AF699070

WITHDRAWN

Alcoholism in the United States

Racial and Ethnic Considerations

Committee on Cultural Psychiatry

Ezra E. H. Griffith, New Haven, CT, *Chairperson*
Henry Chung, New York, NY
Edward Foulks, New Orleans, LA
Francis Lu, San Francisco, CA
Pedro Ruiz, Houston, TX
Ronald Wintrob, Providence, RI
Joe Yamamoto, Los Angeles, CA

Alcoholism in the United States

Racial and Ethnic Considerations

Formulated by the
Committee on Cultural Psychiatry

Group for the Advancement of Psychiatry

Report No. 141

Published by

American Psychiatric Press, Inc.

Washington, DC
London, England

RC
565.6
.M56
A44
1996

Copyright © 1996 Group for the Advancement of Psychiatry
ALL RIGHTS RESERVED
Manufactured in the United States of America on acid-free paper
99 98 97 96 4 3 2 1

Published by American Psychiatric Press, Inc.
1400 K Street, N.W., Washington, DC 20005

Library of Congress Cataloging-in-Publication Data
Alcoholism in the United States : racial and ethnic considerations /
formulated by the Committee on Cultural Psychiatry.
p. cm. — (Report ; no. 141)
Includes bibliographical references.
ISBN 0-87318-209-X
1. Minorities—Alcohol use—United States. 2. Alcoholism—United States—Cross-cultural studies. I. Group for the Advancement of Psychiatry. Committee on Cultural Psychiatry. II. Series: Report (Group for the Advancement of Psychiatry : 1984) ; no. 141.
RC565.6.M56A44 1996
362.29′2′08693—dc20 95-49241
CIP

British Library Cataloguing in Publication Data
A CIP record is available from the British Library.

Contents

Introduction

Alcoholism is a major public health problem in the United States involving great cost in its treatment, as well as lost productivity in the workplace. The total financial impact of alcohol abuse and alcohol dependence is estimated to be about $86 billion each year. Alcohol abuse and dependence are also closely linked to other, costly societal problems, including family disintegration, street crime, and crimes of violence.

There is a widely held belief that alcoholism and its deleterious social consequences are more prevalent among the social/ethnic minority population of the United States than among the majority white population. Another common assumption is that alcohol-related morbidity and mortality are more serious problems in minorities than in whites.

The Committee on Cultural Psychiatry of the Group for the Advancement of Psychiatry set out to check the validity of these and other assumptions about alcohol use, alcohol abuse, alcoholism, and also alcohol abstention in the United States. The committee determined to focus on a review of the scientific literature on these issues in the majority white population, as well as in four of the major racial/ethnic minorities for whom some body of research data exists concerning the issues outlined. The four minority populations to be considered are African American, Hispanic American, Asian American, and Native American (i.e., American Indians and Alaska Natives). Their approximate numbers in the United States population, according to 1990 census figures, are African Americans, 12%; Hispanic Americans, 8%; Asian Americans, 3%; and Native Americans, 1%.

The committee wanted first to delineate the main findings concerning the lifetime prevalence of alcoholism in the majority and minority populations and then outline the prevalence rates for frequent heavy drinking among them, gender differences in these two parameters (lifetime prevalence and heavy drinking), peak risk for alcoholism and heavy alcohol use according to age, and alcohol-related morbidity and mortality. We wanted to make systematic comparisons between minority groups on each of these important issues, as well as compare minority and majority populations along the same lines. We also wanted to examine data on the history of alcoholism in the families of problem drinkers; the relationship between personal and family income and alcoholism; and the effects of urban migration, immigration, and acculturation on alcohol use and abuse. In addition, we wanted to review data on abstinence from alcohol in the majority and minority populations.

Our purpose in undertaking this review was to draw attention to commonalities and differences in all the items listed between the racial/ethnic minority groups and the majority population and then to examine the possible reasons for these similarities and differences, with special attention given to cross-cultural issues.

In addressing the subject of alcohol use and alcohol problems, the committee studied a number of parameters of mental health and social functioning in racial/ethnic minority populations in the United States. These groups represent areas of special research and clinical interest for members of the committee. In this report, the committee did not attempt to apply a specific theoretical formulation in discussing the significance of the findings; instead, the focus is to point out similarities and differences between the groups along the parameters listed; to identify the need for further research that can help clarify the variations between groups and the intragroup factors involved in alcohol use, alcohol abuse, and alcohol abstinence; and finally, to outline the policy implications for treatment and prevention of alcoholism in the designated population groups.

The committee encountered serious difficulties in obtaining alcoholism data prior to 1990 that were based on national rather than regional or even local sampling of the four minority populations. Since that time, some important advances have been made in collecting national census data, particularly in identifying Hispanic Americans and Asian Americans in the 1990 census. The national scope of the National Institute of Mental Health (NIMH)–sponsored Epidemiologic Catchment Area (ECA) study in the 1980s and its inclusion, by design, of an oversampling of both African Americans and Hispanic Americans in several of the ECA study sites have helped overcome previous limitations in alcoholism data for those two important groups. Unfortunately, a comparable approach involving intentional oversampling procedures in collecting alcoholism data for Asian Americans and Native Americans was not included in the ECA study design.

The National Household Health Survey in the 1980s collected valuable alcoholism data on African Americans and Hispanic Americans but again was limited in its sampling of Asian American and Native American families. On the other hand, alcoholism data for all four racial/ethnic populations are included in national mortality statistics and in some national data on disease-related morbidity. Overall, the greatest limitations in national sample data relating to alcohol use and alcoholism apply to the Asian American and Native American groups, as is noted in the chapters devoted to those groups.

The committee is very much aware that the terms *African American, Hispanic American, Asian American,* and *Native American* are descriptive categories that encompass a wide range of population differences within each category and are not mutually exclusive racial/ethnic categories, any more than the category "white" encompasses a homogeneous population. In a country as racially and ethnically diverse as the United States, it would seem self-evident that there is enormous diversity in each of the designated groups: in terms of history of migration to and within the United States, country of origin, genetic features, socioeconomic factors, acculturative stressors, and sociocultural adaptation. All of these distinctions within as well as between groups may influence patterns of alcohol use and abuse, alcohol-related health problems, and alcoholism, as well as treatment and prevention of alcohol-related health and social problems.

Despite the limitations of available alcoholism data and the caveats noted concerning intra- and intergroup comparisons, interesting and sometimes unexpected findings did emerge from the committee's review of the data on alcohol use and alcohol problems in the population groups under study. Those findings are presented in each of the subsequent chapters, which focus in turn on African Americans, Hispanic Americans, Asian Americans, and Native Americans. Each of these chapters includes a brief description of the population, followed by a review of the available literature on lifetime prevalence of alcoholism; frequent heavy drinking; peak risks for alcoholism by age group for both men and women; alcohol abstinence in the population; alcohol-related morbidity and mortality; income and alcohol use; and factors of urban migration, immigration, and acculturation in relation to alcohol use. Intragroup differences are noted and their significance considered. Some issues specific to each population group are also addressed, such as the significance of the flushing response among Asian Americans; religion and religious participation and its relationship to alcohol use; and changes in drinking patterns across generations as a function of acculturative stress, changes in family income, and urban migration.

The report concludes with an overview and summary chapter that draws together common themes and differences in major findings between the minority and majority populations and outlines policy implications for treatment and prevention of alcoholism as well as for needed research related to the majority and minority populations of the United States.

1

Alcohol and African Americans

Alcoholism among African Americans continues to be a topic of substantial interest for several important reasons. First, Rice and colleagues (1) noted that the measurable economic costs of alcohol abuse were high. They pointed out that for 1988, the total fiscal impact of alcohol abuse was about $86 billion, taking into consideration factors such as the loss of productivity caused by alcohol abuse, amounts spent on treatment of alcohol abuse, and indirect costs arising from mortality and morbidity. Given the relatively poor socioeconomic status of African Americans in comparison to whites, one might reasonably speculate that the prevention of alcoholism among African Americans might have a beneficial impact on their socioeconomic status and on their economic productivity.

Second, Otten et al. (2) reminded us that the mortality gap between black and white adult Americans remains impressive. These authors noted that the Secretary's Task Force on Black and Minority Health (3) reported in 1985 that the largest contributors to excess deaths among blacks in comparison to whites were cancer, heart disease and stroke, cirrhosis, diabetes, unintentional injuries, and homicide. The Secretary of Health and Human Services, in a 1987 report (4), reiterated that the incidence of "alcohol-related medical problems, especially liver cirrhosis and cancer of the esophagus, is very high among blacks. Cirrhosis mortality rates for blacks are twice as high as the rates for whites" (4, p. xvii). Therefore, it seems evident that at least to some extent, the problem of alcoholism among African Americans is a matter of life or death.

There are also other elements of interest, such as Franklin's (5) point that at least one study has found a greater risk of fetal alcohol syndrome in infants born to black women than those born to white women. Lex (6) emphasized that some studies have suggested that more blacks than whites have medical complications when being treated for alcoholism. Brown (7) also referred to the dislocation in African American communities that is directly or indirectly linked to chemical dependency. He suggested that alcoholism and drug abuse have some connection to single-parent families, teen pregnancy, family instability, and poor education. These points all argue powerfully for attempting to shed light on the current knowledge we have about alcohol abuse among African Americans and for trying to appreciate the role cultural factors may play in sustaining a level of alcohol abuse that is clearly detrimental to the future of the African American group in the United States. Alcoholism has substantial effects on the morbidity, mortality, and socioeconomic status of African Americans. Understanding why is a challenge of some import.

The 1990 census estimate put the African American population at about 12% (30 million people) of the United States resident population of 249 million people (8). However, Brown (7) stated that there is no monolithic African American community and that African Americans include individuals from different countries and cultures. Consequently, African American communities may differ in the degree to which they tolerate alcohol consumption or abuse. This variability in the African American community may increase if one considers the potential impact of the growing number of blacks who are the products of interracial marriages.

Rates and Trends of Alcoholism Among African Americans

Epidemiologic Catchment Area Program

Overall rates. The National Institute of Mental Health (NIMH) Epidemiologic Catchment Area (ECA) program carried out community surveys at five different United States sites in the early 1980s. Using DSM-III (9) criteria, the program reported lifetime prevalence rates of alcoholism among blacks (10). These data showed little difference in the total lifetime rates between blacks (23.7% for men, 5% for women) and whites (23.4% for men, 4.5% for women). When broken down by age, however, some pattern differences did emerge, as can be seen in

Table 1–1. For example, the rates for white men peaked in the young adult age group (18–29 years) and then progressively decreased. In contrast, the rates for black men started at 12.6% in the 18–29 age group, increased sharply in the 30–44 age group, peaked in the 45–64 age group, and then decreased. Women in both races show substantially lower rates than their male counterparts, with white women following the trend of white men, and black women following the trend of black men.

Urban/rural patterns. Blazer and colleagues (11) used the ECA data (in this case, 6-month prevalence rates) for Durham, North Carolina, to examine certain assumptions generally made about drinking patterns. These assumptions were as follows:

- Urban settings may predispose individuals to increased alcohol-related problems.
- Young working women located in urban settings may be especially vulnerable to alcohol abuse.

Table 1–1. Lifetime prevalence of alcoholism (Epidemiologic Catchment Area study, 1980–1981, five sites)

Age group (years)	Whites (%)	Blacks (%)
18–29		
Men	28.31	12.61
Women	7.50	4.19
30–44		
Men	27.00	31.33
Women	5.47	6.88
45–64		
Men	19.75	32.99
Women	2.60	7.33
Over 65		
Men	12.53	21.63
Women	1.46	2.20
Total		
Men	23.44	23.71
Women	4.52	5.47

Source. Adapted from Helzer JE, Burnam A, McEvory LT: "Alcohol Abuse and Dependence," in *Psychiatric Disorders in America.* Edited by Robins LN, Regier DA. New York, Free Press, 1991, pp. 81–115.

- Rural alcohol use may be better tolerated than urban use.
- Rural regions often report lower rates of alcoholism than urban sites.

The results showed that rural black men were more likely than urban black men to have alcoholism in all age groups. This finding was not duplicated in a robust fashion for white men or for women of either race. In a discussion of their findings, the authors raised several possible explanations:

- Given the partial hereditary explanation of alcoholism, intermarriage among rural blacks might account for the rise in alcoholism rates among rural blacks.
- Poverty and isolation may be especially harsh among rural blacks.
- There may be reverse drift among black alcoholic patients from urban to rural communities.
- Rural blacks may complain more about alcoholism.
- Rural blacks may in fact drink more.

Female patterns. Lillie-Blanton and colleagues (12) used the ECA program data for the Baltimore, Maryland, site to describe differences in alcohol use among black and white women. There were significant differences in the study sample on the basis of age, income, education, and marital status. Black women were younger, less formally educated, and of lower economic status; they were also less likely to be married. The authors made it clear these sociodemographic differences were to be considered in commenting on the study's results. The lifetime prevalence rates of alcoholism for Baltimore showed the same pattern as that found for the five sites overall. In other words, black female rates increased progressively until age 60 and then decreased. (Note that in this study, the age categories were slightly different from those cited for the five-site results.) Black women had a somewhat higher lifetime prevalence rate of alcoholism than white women (6% vs. 3%), but the current prevalence rates were not considered to be distinctly dissimilar (blacks, 3%; whites, 2%).

The authors also used categorical titles to describe the women's drinking, such as *nondrinker* and *heavy drinker* (12). A nondrinker consumed zero ounces of absolute alcohol per day, and a heavy drinker used one or more ounces of absolute alcohol per day, or about two cans of beer or two drinks of wine or other liquor per day. The authors showed that the drinking patterns of black and white women were similar. About 48% of blacks and 40% of whites reported no drinking in the month preceding the interview, and the percentage of heavy drinkers among the black (5%) and white (4%) women was also similar. Table 1–2 shows that the percentage of black women nondrinkers in each group was larger than that of white women nondrinkers. The authors found that the contrasts were most significant for young women (ages 18–24) and for those over age 60. The percentage of heavy drinkers peaked at a later age (45–59 years) for black women than for white women (25–44 years) and then decreased in both groups. Notably, there were no heavy drinkers among black women over age 60.

After performing correlation analyses, the authors concluded that about the same percentage of black and white women in this study had an alcohol use disorder, but there were racial differences regarding the likelihood of nondrinking and heavy drinking that resulted from the effects of sociodemographic characteristics. Young black women (18–24 years) and older black women (over age 60) were more likely to be nondrinkers in comparison to white women, and those with less than 12 years of formal education were more likely to be nondrinkers than those with more education. Among heavy drinkers, there was a similar percentage of black and white women who had not completed high school. However, black women with more than 12 years of education were less likely than white women of similar education to be heavy drinkers.

Lillie-Blanton et al. (12) therefore argued that racial differences in alcohol-related morbidity and mortality among women cannot be ascribed to differences in drinking patterns, but differences should be sought in later detection of symptoms, less-effective treatment techniques, or the coexistence of other diseases.

Table 1–2. Percentages of women in selected drinking groups by race (weighted data, Baltimore Epidemiologic Catchment Area site)

	Nondrinkers		Heavy drinkers	
Age (years)	**Black**	**White**	**Black**	**White**
18–24	44.3	26.3	3.5	3.5
25–44	33.9	24.7	6.2	5.2
45–59	57.9	44.3	8.8	4.7
60 +	83.1	55.8	0.0	3.3

Source. Adapted from Lillie-Blanton ML, MacKenzie E, Anthony JC: "Black-White Differences in Alcohol Use by Women: Baltimore Survey Findings." *Public Health Reports* 106:124–133, 1991.

Amaro et al. (13), in an article predating the work by Lillie-Blanton et al., cited the repeated early finding that the prevalence and consequences of alcohol abuse are higher and more severe among black than among white women. Clearly, the Baltimore study challenges those findings. Amaro et al. additionally noted the puzzle reflected in the findings that serious alcohol problems are found at a later age in black women, yet black women seemed to enter treatment earlier than white women. In their own study of a small cohort, Amaro et al. (13) confirmed that the black women in treatment were significantly younger than white counterparts. They also found that black alcoholic women in the study were more likely than white women to report feelings of social isolation and not to have access to third-party coverage for alcoholism treatment.

1984 National Survey

In 1990, Herd (14) described some essential findings from a 1984 national survey regarding drinking patterns among the United States black population. She thought the study important because of conflicting notions about black alcoholism. For example, some studies suggested that drinking and drunkenness were common among blacks, whereas other studies showed that a comparatively higher percentage of blacks were abstainers in comparison to whites, and rates of heavy alcohol use were similar for whites and blacks.

The study was based on data gathered through personal interviews with 723 black and 743 white men who were representative of the general American black and white population. In the samples, the black men were younger, more likely to have household incomes below $10,000, more likely to be unemployed, and more likely than the white men to be divorced or separated or never married.

Results showed that black and white men had similar drinking patterns, with blacks having a slightly higher rate of abstainers (29% vs. 24%) and slightly lower rate of frequent heavy drinkers (15% vs. 19%) than whites. Patterned differences did emerge, however, when the data were analyzed as a function of age, as seen in Table 1–3. Among the frequent heavy drinker group, the rate for whites in the 18- to 29-year age group was considerably higher than that for blacks. The rates for blacks remained fairly stable, peaked in the 50- to 59-year age group, and then dropped. The white rate peaked in the 18- to 29-year age group and then declined with increasing age. In those younger than 50, the rate for blacks was lower than that for whites. Table 1–3 also shows that the rate of abstainers among both blacks and whites peaked in the over-60 age group. The rate

Table 1–3. Percentages of men in selected drinking groups by race (weighted data, 1984 National Household Health Survey)

Age (years)	Abstainers		Frequent heavy drinkers	
	Black	White	Black	White
18–29	23	17	16	31
30–39	15	13	17	21
40–49	37	21	14	19
50–59	29	30	20	17
60 +	60	41	5	4

Source. Adapted from Herd D: "Subgroup Differences in Drinking Patterns Among Black and White Men: Results From a National Survey." *Journal of Studies on Alcohol* 51:221–232, 1990.

of black male abstainers was somewhat higher than that of white abstainers in almost every age group.

When the data were analyzed as a function of family income, Herd (14) found that among white men, the rates of frequent heavy drinking were very high among the poorest men (income < $6,000), dropped for men earning between $6,000 and $10,000 a year, and then increased as income increased. Among white men, then, the highest levels of alcohol drinking occurred in those earning the most money. In contrast, among black men, the heaviest drinking occurred in the middle income group. The poorest and the richest black men did not engage much in frequent heavy drinking.

After performing log-linear analysis of the data, Herd found certain patterns persisted. Young white men showed higher rates of heavier drinking than middle-age or older whites; young blacks drank less heavily than middle-age blacks; black men in the highest income brackets showed lower rates of heavier drinking than blacks at low or moderate income levels; and the income differences for white men appeared to be smaller and to be overshadowed by age.

Corresponding data for women have been reported from the 1984 National Household Health Survey performed by the U.S. Department of Health and Human Services (15). These data in aggregate showed a higher rate of abstainers among black women (46%) than among white women (34%) but with relatively little difference between the rate of heavy drinking in black women (4%) and that in white women (5%). Table 1–4 shows the data broken down by age. There are proportionately more black women

Table 1–4. Percentages of women in selected drinking groups by race (weighted data, 1984 National Household Health Survey)

	Abstainers		Frequent heavy drinkers	
Age (years)	**Black**	**White**	**Black**	**White**
18–29	34	22	6	7
30–39	32	30	5	8
40–49	56	35	6	7
50–59	60	35	2	1
60 +	69	49	1	1

Source. Adapted from U.S. Department of Health and Human Services: *Health Status of Minorities and Low Income Groups*, 3rd Edition. Washington, DC, U.S. Government Printing Office, 1991.

abstainers than white women abstainers in every age category, and number of abstainers progressively increased with age in both groups. With regard to frequent heavy drinking, there is relatively little difference between black and white women, and the rate of heavy drinking in women is substantially lower than that of men, seen in Table 1–3.

Alcohol-Related Mortality

Mortality data are commonly used to estimate certain effects of alcoholism on population groups. Such data are to be used with caution because reporting bias has been invoked as a reason for some of the differences noted. For example, it has been suggested that physicians may be less likely to report that deaths of whites were related to alcohol. Table 1–5 reflects data obtained from the January 1993 *Monthly Vital Statistics Report* (16). The category of alcohol-induced causes of death includes deaths from dependent and nondependent use of alcohol but excludes accidents, homicides, and other causes indirectly related to alcohol use; in this category, the rate for the black population is about 2.6 times the rate for the white population. Deaths from chronic liver disease and cirrhosis are highest among the black male population. An indirect index of alcoholism, such as homicide, shows that black men are the most prominent bearers of this form of death.

Discussion

Because this commentary relies distinctly on epidemiological studies, it is useful to recall important reservations that have been stated about

Table 1–5. Age-adjusted death rates per 100,000 population for certain conditions by race and sex, United States, 1990

	White			Black		
Conditions	**Both sexes**	**Men**	**Women**	**Both sexes**	**Men**	**Women**
Alcohol-induced causes	6.2	9.9	2.8	16.1	26.6	7.7
Chronic liver disease, cirrhosis	10.3	13.6	7.1	12.3	16.6	8.5
Malignancies of digestive organs	49.6	53.4	46	49	55.5	43.2
Motor vehicle accidents	19.0	26.7	11.6	18.2	28.1	9.4
Homicide and legal intervention	5.8	9.0	2.8	39.8	69.2	13.5

Source. *Monthly Vital Statistics Report* 41(suppl 7):28, 29, 38, 1993.

these data. For example, Brown (7) argued that the epidemiological surveys may have been hampered by underrepresentation of African Americans. He explained how surveys of high school students would probably not have covered African American dropouts, among whom one might expect a significantly elevated level of alcohol and drug abuse. In addition, data from hospitals and medical examiners were too variable to be considered solidly reliable. Finally, Brown suggested that it was difficult to be sure how any study cohort of African Americans compared ethnographically to the actual community from which the sample was drawn.

With these reservations in mind, it is helpful to summarize the main points of the data reviewed here on alcohol abuse among African Americans. These data show

- There is little difference between African Americans and whites in the lifetime prevalence of alcoholism.
- White and African American women show substantially lower prevalence rates than their male counterparts.
- The prevalence of alcoholism among African Americans is greatest in middle age.
- The alcoholism prevalence for African Americans is low in the young adult group and then increases, in contrast to the alcoholism

prevalence for whites, which starts at a moderately high level in the young adult group and then decreases.

- Among men, blacks show a consistently higher level of abstainers than whites.
- Among women, blacks show a consistently higher level of abstainers than whites.
- Findings in one geographic area in the South suggest that rural black men in all age groups are more likely than their urban counterparts to have alcoholism.
- Overall heavy drinking among black and white women appears to be similar.
- Overall heavy drinking among black and white men appears to be similar.
- Deaths from alcohol-induced causes are about 2.5 times higher in the black population than in the white population.
- Deaths from chronic liver disease and cirrhosis are somewhat higher among blacks than among whites.

It is surprising that the lifetime prevalence rates for alcoholism are similar for African Americans and whites, given the finding that deaths from alcohol-induced causes are higher for African Americans than for whites. Indeed, these higher mortality rates commonly lead clinicians to think that blacks abuse alcohol more often than whites. However, this is not the case, and the question remains as to what factors possibly account for the difference in mortality between the two groups resulting from alcohol-induced causes.

It is possible that poverty and poor education interact in some way to account for the mortality difference. For example, those blacks who do drink heavily are likely to have poor nutritional status, which in turn exacerbates the negative effects of alcohol. These same black drinkers may have more limited access to health care than whites or may make use of health care at a later time in the evolution of their health problems. It is also possible that blacks detect their symptoms of disease later than do whites and so seek health care when their alcohol-related diseases are more advanced.

Alternatively, blacks may show symptoms of alcoholism later than whites do, or treatment techniques may be less effective in blacks than in whites. It is also possible that disorders that complicate the treatment of alcoholism and result in medical or neurological comorbidity are seen more frequently in African American drinkers than in white drinkers.

There is no good evidence at this time that would lead us to conclude that standard treatment techniques are less effective in blacks than in others, although such treatment interventions are likely to need modification when applied to certain subpopulations. For example, with multiproblem individuals, greater efforts in the form of case management, alcohol-free housing, and vocational rehabilitation may be necessary.

Although these factors may partially explain the significant mortality among blacks that derives from alcohol abuse, the similarity of lifetime prevalence rates among blacks and white remains puzzling. Brown (7) delineated several factors that might explain patterns of African American drinking. Among these were unemployment/underemployment, inadequate education, criminality, poverty, family disorganization, availability of alcoholic beverage retail outlets in the black community, legitimization of alcohol consumption in the black community, tolerated behaviors among black adolescent consumers of alcohol, and existence of functional rites of passage in the black community that use alcohol as an important element of the ritual. In fact, a careful reading of Brown's argument would suggest that his position is difficult to defend. The factors he has cited would normally be expected to underscore high prevalence rates of alcohol abuse.

For example, family disorganization, inadequate education, criminality, and poverty would be expected to be powerfully felt by adolescent African Americans, who then would manifest their frustration in violence and alcohol abuse. As we have shown, black adolescents abstain more and show less frequent heavy drinking than their white counterparts. This is a significant point and shows that important fundamental research remains to be done to resolve this dilemma. In addition, black adolescents are usually expected to bear the brunt of homicide, suicide, and substance abuse. It is intriguing that this pattern is not replicated through the alcohol abuse data. It is also not clear why frequent heavy drinking among black men peaks in middle age, in contrast to whites, who show the peak much earlier. The emergence of this vulnerability to alcohol so late in the individual life cycle makes one wonder what biological and sociopsychological factors come together at that point in time to push black men to use alcohol as a coping mechanism or to engage in its abuse. Another important question is whether some young African Americans not abusing alcohol may, in fact, be abusing other substances such as marijuana and heroin or cocaine.

We cannot really be sure that alcohol and drug use affect the same subgroups of the African American population. Even if that were the case, it is not clear what factors would support the preference of cocaine, for example, over alcohol. It may be that crack cocaine's success in the minority inner-city population is caused mainly by its wide availability and aggressive marketing by suppliers of the drug. It may also be that the powerful stimulant effects of cocaine enhance the inner-city individual's capacity to contend with all the social, economic, and psychological problems posed by the urban environment. Conversely, it may be that those who maintain the struggle in the adolescent and young adult years then gradually shift to preferring the numbing effects of alcohol. In both cases, of course, cocaine and alcohol still have devastating effects on the families of the abusers.

Two other important findings worth noting are the lower rates of alcohol abuse among black women in comparison to black men and the higher rates of alcohol abuse among rural black men in North Carolina in comparison to their urban compatriots. Why black women continue to be relatively protected against the ravages of alcohol in comparison to black men is still a puzzle. The traditional arguments that black men experience racism and oppression more than black women are no longer acceptable, because the roles of black women are clearer and better understood. The black woman's task in holding together her family and ensuring the family's economic viability cannot seriously be argued to be less arduous than the black man's role. However, it is nevertheless possible that the use of alcohol as a coping mechanism remains a more acceptable social possibility for men than for women. This possibility of greater cultural acceptance was posited by Blazer and colleagues (11) as one way to explain the higher rates of alcoholism among rural blacks in North Carolina in comparison to their urban counterparts, although a single factor cannot explain this difference.

This leaves us with the obvious conclusion that substantial work needs to be done to elucidate the patterns of alcoholism currently found among African Americans. This is a complex task that invokes the need for a serious, coherent, interdisciplinary effort at understanding the many roles played by alcohol in an African American national community that is fractious and subject to the vagaries of education, socioeconomic status, and other characteristics. Particular attention must be paid to the elucidation of the puzzling phenomenon of young men's apparent dislike for alcohol in comparison to an apparent preference for drugs such as cocaine. Greater focus also must be applied to the effect of parental alcoholism on the family's function and on the children growing up in these dysfunctional families.

References

1. Rice DP, Kelman S, Miller LS: The economic cost of alcohol abuse. Alcohol Health Res World 15:307–316, 1991
2. Otten MW, Teutsch SM, Williamson DF, et al: The effect of known risk factors on the excess mortality of black adults in the United States. JAMA 263:845–850, 1990
3. Report of the Secretary's Task Force on Black and Minority Health. Washington, DC, U.S. Department of Health and Human Services, August 1985
4. Sixth Special Report to the U.S. Congress on Alcohol and Health From the Secretary of Health and Human Services. Washington, DC, U.S. Department of Health and Human Services, January 1987
5. Franklin JE Jr: Alcoholism among blacks. Hosp Community Psychiatry 40:1120–1127, 1989
6. Lex BW: Review of alcohol problems in ethnic minority groups. J Consult Clin Psychol 55:293–300, 1987
7. Brown LS Jr: Alcohol abuse prevention in African-American communities. J Natl Med Assoc 85:665–673, 1993
8. U.S. Bureau of the Census: Statistical Abstract of the United States: 1992, 112th Edition. Washington, DC, U.S. Government Printing Office, 1992
9. American Psychiatric Association: Diagnostic and Statistical Manual of Mental Disorders, 3rd Edition. Washington, DC, American Psychiatric Association, 1980
10. Helzer JE, Burnam A, McEvory LT: Alcohol abuse and dependence, in Psychiatric Disorders in America. Edited by Robins LN, Regier DA. New York, Free Press, 1991, pp 81–115
11. Blazer D, Crowell BA Jr, George LK: Alcohol abuse and dependence in the rural south. Arch Gen Psychiatry 44:736–740, 1987
12. Lillie-Blanton M, MacKenzie E, Anthony JC: Black-white differences in alcohol use by women: Baltimore survey findings. Public Health Rep 106:124–133, 1991
13. Amaro H, Beckman LJ, Mays VM: A comparison of black and white women entering alcoholism treatment. J Stud Alcohol 48:220–228, 1987
14. Herd D: Subgroup differences in drinking patterns among black and white men: results from a national survey. J Stud Alcohol 51:221–232, 1990
15. U.S. Department of Health and Human Services: Health Status of Minorities and Low Income Groups, 3rd Edition. Washington, DC, U.S. Government Printing Office, 1991
16. Monthly Vital Statistics Report 41 (suppl 7):28–38, 1993

2

Alcohol and Hispanic Americans

The previous chapter reminded us that African Americans are not a homogeneous group of people. That reminder is even more relevant as we consider the use and abuse of alcohol among Hispanic Americans, who come from multiple geographic areas and bring with them a variety of differing subcultures. Still, traditional use makes reference to Hispanic Americans as though they are a single entity.

Hispanic Americans represent about 8.4% of the United States population, or about 20.7 million people (1). Mexican Americans are the largest subgroup of Hispanic Americans (64%, or 13.3 million); Puerto Ricans are next, at 10.5%, or 2.2 million; and Cuban Americans follow, at 4.9%, or 1 million. These numbers do not include illegal aliens or Puerto Ricans residing in Puerto Rico.

The available data on alcoholism among Hispanic Americans do not permit any further differentiation of subgroups. Nevertheless, it is well known that some United States cities have significant numbers of Hispanic Americans from Caribbean, Central American, and South American countries.

In this chapter we present the data from the large Epidemiologic Catchment Area (ECA) study and other relevant small-scale studies on alcoholism among Hispanic Americans. We also advance some hypotheses to explain the major trends in the data.

Rates and Trends of Alcoholism Among Hispanic Americans

ECA Program: Overall Rates

The national ECA study included data from five survey sites (2). The results of this study, as seen in Table 2–1, show that the total lifetime prevalence rates of alcoholism were higher among Hispanic American men than among white men (30.02% vs. 23.44%). However, the total rate of alcoholism was slightly lower among Hispanic American women than among white women (3.85% vs. 4.52%). In terms of age differences, alcoholism among Hispanic American men peaked in those age 30–44 years (35.91%), whereas the peak for white men occurred in those age 18–29 years (28.31%). In white men, the rates of alcoholism progressively decreased as age increased. For Hispanic American women, alcoholism peaked in those age 18–29 years (4.90%) and then progressively decreased. White women fol-

Table 2–1. Lifetime prevalence of alcoholism (Epidemiologic Catchment Area Study, 1980–1981, five sites)

Age group (years)	Hispanic Americans (%)	Whites (%)
18–29		
Men	29.76	28.31
Women	4.90	7.50
30–44		
Men	35.91	27.00
Women	3.67	5.47
45–64		
Men	25.97	19.75
Women	3.46	2.60
Over 65		
Men	18.10	12.53
Women	0.79	1.46
Total		
Men	30.02	23.44
Women	3.85	4.52

Source. Adapted from Helzer JE, Burnam A, McEvoy LT: "Alcohol Abuse and Dependence," in *Psychiatric Disorders in America.* Edited by Robins LN, Reigier DA. New York, Free Press, 1991, pp. 81–115.

lowed the pattern of white men, with alcoholism peaking in those age 18–29 years (7.50%) and then progressively decreasing. In Table 2–1, it is also important to note that the rates of alcoholism among Hispanic American men were higher than the rates of alcoholism among white men in every age category. However, the rates of alcoholism for Hispanic American women were lower than the rates of alcoholism for white women in every age category, with the exception of the 45- to 64-year age group, in which the rate for Hispanic American women was higher than that for white women (3.46% vs. 2.60%).

1984 National Household Health Survey

This survey, done in 1984 (3) and summarized in Table 2–2, shows, at a national level, the pattern of abstention and frequent heavy drinking

Table 2–2. Drinking patterns (1984 National Household Health Survey)

	Abstainers (%)		Frequent heavy drinkers (%)	
Age group (years)	**Men**	**Women**	**Men**	**Women**
18–29				
Hispanic Americans	22	40	17	2
Whites	17	22	31	7
30–39				
Hispanic Americans	17	45	26	2
Whites	13	30	21	8
40–49				
Hispanic Americans	23	41	11	2
Whites	21	35	19	7
50–59				
Hispanic Americans	24	47	12	8
Whites	30	35	17	1
Over 60				
Hispanic Americans	30	78	3	0
Whites	41	49	4	1
Total				
Hispanic Americans	22	47	17	3
Whites	24	34	19	5

Source. Adapted from U.S. Department of Health and Human Services: *Health Status of Minorities and Low Income Groups*, 3rd Edition. Washington, DC, U.S. Government Printing Office, 1991, p. 264.

among Hispanic Americans and whites. In terms of frequent heavy drinking, the peak for Hispanic American men was in the 30- to 39-year age group (26%), whereas the peak for white men was in the 18- to 29-year age group (31%), with a subsequent progressive decrease with age. However, the pattern for women was quite different. The peak for Hispanic American women was in the 50- to 59-year age group (8%), whereas for white women, the 18- to 29-year age group (7%), the 30- to 39-year age group (8%), and the 40- to 49-year age group (7%) had practically the same rates, which then decreased sharply in the 50- to 59-year age group. The total rate of frequent heavy drinking was relatively similar for Hispanic American men (17%) and white men (19%). Hispanic American women (3%) and white women (5%) also had similar overall rates.

On examining differences in the various age categories, we see that the rates of frequent heavy drinking were higher among white men than among Hispanic American men in every age category, with the exception of the 30- to 39-year age group, in which the rate was higher among Hispanic American men (26% vs. 21%). Also, the comparison of the rates of frequent heavy drinking among women shows that the rates for white women were higher in every age category than those for Hispanic American women, with the exception of the rates in the 50- to 59-year age group, in which the rate for Hispanic American women was higher than that for white women (8% vs. 1%).

Regarding the rates of abstainers, the total rates were quite similar between Hispanic American men and white men (22% vs. 24%). However, Hispanic American men abstained more than white men in the early years (ages 18–49) but less in the later years (ages 50 and above). Among women, the rates of abstention were higher among Hispanic American women than among white women in every age category, and this was also reflected in the figures for total rates (47% vs. 34%).

ECA Program: Los Angeles Site

As part of the national ECA study (4), surveys were carried out in Los Angeles, California. This local study, as shown in Table 2–3, focused on the lifetime prevalence rates of alcohol disorders among Mexican Americans and whites. The highest rates occurred in the 30- to 39-year age group for Mexican American men (37.3%) and in the 40- to 49-year age group for white men (24.1%). Alcoholism rates varied little among all age categories for white men ages 18–49, then decreased somewhat. There was more variation in alcoholism rates among white women. Rates dropped sharply

Table 2–3. Lifetime prevalence of alcohol disorders (Epidemiologic Catchment Area Study, 1980–1982, Los Angeles)

Age group (years)	Mexican Americans (%)	Whites (%)
18–29		
Men	30.5	22.2
Women	5.4	11.7
30–39		
Men	37.3	21.7
Women	3.9	9.7
40–49		
Men	26.2	24.1
Women	7.0	13.8
Over 50		
Men	33.4	17.8
Women	2.4	4.8

Source. Adapted from Burnam MA: "Prevalence of Alcohol and Dependence Among Mexican-Americans and Non-Hispanic Whites in the Community," in *Alcohol Use Among U.S. Ethnic Minorities* (Research Monograph No 18). Edited by Spiegler D, Tate D, Aitken S, et al (DHHS Publ No ADM-89-1435). Washington, DC, U.S. Government Printing Office, 1989, pp. 163–177.

for women over age 50, as was the case for white men. Comparison of the two groups shows that the rates for Mexican American men were higher than those of white men in every age category. However, for women the opposite was true—that is, the rates for Mexican American women were lower than those for white women in every age category.

Hispanic Health and Nutrition Examination Survey

In addition to studying a series of illnesses/conditions, this study (5) also focused on the alcoholism pattern among some of the major Hispanic American subgroups residing in the United States. Specifically, the survey dealt with the pattern of abstention and frequent heavy drinking among Mexican Americans, Puerto Ricans, and Cuban Americans. The results of this study were summarized in the National Clearinghouse for Alcohol and Drug Information (6), as shown in Table 2–4.

With regard to frequent heavy drinking among men, Mexican Americans led the group with a rate of 15.3%, followed by Puerto Ricans with

Table 2–4. Hispanic American drinking patterns (HHANES data, 1982–1984)

Subgroup	Abstainers (%)	Frequent heavy drinkers (%)
Mexican Americans		
(*N* = 4,590)		
Men	32.3	15.3
Women	68.5	1.4
Total	50.3	8.4
Puerto Ricans		
(*N* = 1,821)		
Men	42.6	13.0
Women	71.2	2.3
Total	59.6	6.7
Cuban Americans		
(*N* = 1,060)		
Men	37.8	7.9
Women	78.2	0.4
Total	59.8	3.8

Source. Adapted from *Alcohol, Drug Abuse and Mental Health Administration: National Clearinghouse for Alcohol and Drug Information, Update.* January 1989, p. 2.

13%, and Cuban Americans with 7.9%. Puerto Ricans, however, had the highest level of female frequent heavy drinking (2.3%), followed by Mexican Americans with 1.4%, and Cuban Americans with 0.4%. These women's rates are quite low, and differences among them may not have much significance. As a total group, Mexican Americans had the highest rate of frequent heavy drinking (8.4%), followed by Puerto Ricans with 6.7%, and Cuban Americans with 3.8%.

The figures for abstainers among men show that Puerto Ricans led the group with 42.6%, followed by Cuban Americans with 37.8%, and Mexican Americans with 32.3%. Rates for female abstainers were highest among Cuban Americans (78.2%), followed by Puerto Ricans (71.2%) and Mexican Americans (68.5%). As a total group, however, Mexican Americans abstained less (50.3%) than Cuban Americans and Puerto Ricans, who had similar levels of abstention (59.8% and 59.6%, respectively). In summary, as a group, Mexican Americans abstained less and drank more, whereas Cuban Americans abstained more and drank less.

Other Studies

Other studies have considered the relationship between Hispanic American drinking patterns and income, educational levels, acculturation, and migration. The first study, summarized in Table 2–5, assessed the interaction between income levels and the rates of abstention and frequent heavy drinking (7). For Hispanic American women, the rates for frequent heavy drinking were so low that the correlation with income seemed tenuous. However, abstinence seemed to decrease as income increased. For Hispanic American men, the level of frequent heavy drinking increased as income levels increased, and the level of abstention decreased with increasing income, with the exception of that in the $20,001–30,000 income bracket.

In comparing educational levels and alcoholism rates, the same study, as shown in Table 2–6, demonstrated that the abstention rates for Hispanic American men and women with some college education were much lower than the rates for individuals with only a high school or elementary school education. The rates for frequent heavy drinking were higher among Hispanic American men with some college education than among men with a high school or elementary school education. Among Hispanic American women, the rates for frequent heavy drinking were too low to be differentiated significantly.

Another study (8) compared acculturation levels and alcoholism. This study, as demonstrated in Table 2–7, showed that the rates of daily

Table 2–5. Income and Hispanic American drinking patterns (national sample, $N = 1{,}453$)

	Abstainers (%)		Frequent heavy drinkers (%)	
Income	**Men**	**Women**	**Men**	**Women**
Up to $6,000	24	67	10	2
$6,000 to $10,000	19	58	14	2
$10,001 to $15,000	18	49	14	1
$15,001 to $20,000	13	44	11	3
$20,001 to $30,000	43	29	15	5
Over $30,000	4	22	30	3

Source. Adapted from Caetano R: "Drinking Patterns and Alcohol Problems in a National Sample of U.S. Hispanics," in *Alcohol Use Among U.S. Ethnic Minorities* (Research Monograph No 18). Edited by Spiegler D, Tate D, Aitken S, et al (DHSS Publ No ADM-89-1435). Washington, DC, U.S. Government Printing Office, 1989, pp. 147–162.

Table 2–6. Education and Hispanic American drinking patterns (national sample, $N = 1{,}453$)

Education	Abstainers (%) Men	Abstainers (%) Women	Frequent heavy drinkers (%) Men	Frequent heavy drinkers (%) Women
Up to 8th grade	32	59	16	0
Grammar school	47	73	13	3
High school	19	39	11	1
Some college	11	26	32	2

Source. Adapted from Caetano R: "Drinking Patterns and Alcohol Problems in a National Sample of U.S. Hispanics," in *Alcohol Use Among U.S. Ethnic Minorities* (Research Monograph No 18). Edited by Spiegler D, Tate D, Aitken S, et al (DHSS Publ No ADM-89-1435). Washington, DC, U.S. Government Printing Office, 1989, pp. 147–162.

drinking among Mexican American men increased significantly with each generation. However, the opposite was true for Mexican American women. Monthly drinking rates for both Mexican American men and Mexican American women decreased with subsequent generations.

The patterns of migration as related to alcoholism were studied by Caetano and Medina Mora (9). As shown in Table 2–8, this study compared rates of abstention and frequent heavy drinkers among Mexicans, Mexican American migrants, and United States–born Mexican Americans. The rate of frequent heavy drinking in Mexican men (6%) was lower than that in recently arrived Mexican migrant men (27%) and in

Table 2–7. Acculturation and drinking patterns among Mexicans and Mexican Americans (national sample, $N = 1{,}453$)

Acculturation level	Daily (%) Men	Daily (%) Women	Monthly (%) Men	Monthly (%) Women
Mexicans	13	6	56	91
Mexican Americans				
First generation	20	7	34	76
Second generation	21	3	24	59
Third generation	38	4	11	48

Source. Adapted from Gilbert MJ: "Alcohol-Related Practices, Problems, and Norms Among Mexican Americans: an Overview," in *Alcohol Use Among U.S. Ethnic Minorities* (Research Monograph No 18). Edited by Spiegler D, Tate D, Aitken S, et al (DHHS Publ No ADM-89-1435). Washington, DC, U.S. Government Printing Office, 1989, pp. 115–134.

Table 2–8. Alcoholism among Mexicans, Mexican migrants, and Mexican Americans

Group	Abstainers (%) Men	Abstainers (%) Women	Frequent heavy drinkers (%) Men	Frequent heavy drinkers (%) Women
Mexicans (Michoacan)	26	66	6	1
Mexican migrants (1–5 years)	17	70	27	0
United States–born Mexican Americans	33	33	9	2

Source. Adapted from Caetano R, Medina Mora ME: "Acculturation and Drinking Among People of Mexican Descent in Mexico and the United States." *Journal of Studies on Alcohol* 49(5):462–471, 1988.

United States–born Mexican Americans (9%). However, for women, the rates of frequent heavy drinking were similar among all groups. In addition, the rates of frequent heavy drinking were lower among women than among men in all groups.

The rate of abstention in Mexican men (26%) was lower than that in United States–born Mexican American men (33%) but higher than that in recently arrived Mexican migrant men (17%). For women abstainers, the opposite was true. Mexican women's rate of abstention (66%) was higher than that of United States–born Mexican American women (33%) but lower than that of recently arrived Mexican migrant women (70%).

Alcohol-Related Morbidity

Burnam (4) compared alcohol-related morbidity among Mexican Americans and whites. As shown in Table 2–9, the rates of arrests, "the shakes," pancreatitis, and liver disease were higher in white men than in Mexican American men. The rates for blackouts were similar in both groups. The rates of arrests, blackouts, "the shakes," and pancreatitis were higher in white women than in Mexican American women. However, the opposite was true for liver disease. Mexican American women had higher rates for liver diseases than white women. Gender comparisons in both ethnic groups show that the rate of arrests was higher among men than among women. However, the rates of "the shakes" and pancreatitis were higher among women than men. Also, the rate of liver disease was higher among Mexican American women than among Mexican American men.

Table 2–9. Alcohol-related problems among persons with alcoholism (Epidemiologic Catchment Area Study, 1980–1982, Los Angeles)

	Men (%)		Women (%)	
Problems	**Mexican Americans**	**Whites**	**Mexican Americans**	**Whites**
Arrests	29.8	33.9	6.5	20.2
Blackouts	50.0	49.5	49.2	66.4
"The shakes"	18.0	26.6	23.7	27.9
Pancreatitis	1.4	13.8	10.3	21.2
Liver disease	1.6	4.7	8.5	4.8

Source. Adapted from Burnam MA: "Prevalence of Alcohol Abuse and Dependence Among Mexican Americans and Non-Hispanic Whites in the Community," in *Alcohol Use Among U.S. Ethnic Minorities* (Research Monograph No 18). Edited by Spiegler D, Tate D, Aitken S, et al (DHHS Publ No ADM-89-1435). Washington, DC, U.S. Government Printing Office, 1989, pp. 163–177.

Summary of the Findings

The following conclusions seem merited from a review of the studies mentioned above:

1. Hispanic American men drink more during their young adult and early middle-age years.
2. Hispanic American women drink more during their young adult and middle-age years.
3. Hispanic American men drink more than Hispanic American women regardless of age.
4. Frequent heavy drinking peaks at age 30–39 years in Hispanic American men and at age 50–59 years in Hispanic American women.
5. Mexican American men drink more and abstain less than either Puerto Rican or Cuban American men.
6. Hispanic American men and women drink more as their income increases.
7. Hispanic American women abstain less as their income increases.
8. Hispanic American men and women abstain less as their educational level increases.
9. Mexican-born men drink less on a daily basis than Mexican American men.
10. The amount of daily drinking increases from generation to generation for Mexican American men but decreases for women.

11. Mexican American migrant men who have recently arrived in the United States drink more than Mexican American men who have resided in the United States more than 5 years and United States–born Mexican American men.
12. Mexican American migrant women who have recently arrived in the United States abstain more than Mexican American women who have resided in the United States more than 5 years or United States–born Mexican American women.
13. Mexican American women are more affected with alcohol-related pancreatitis and liver diseases than are Mexican American men.

Discussion

It is worth considering first the finding that Hispanic American men tend to drink more than white men. It is possible that the commonly cited Hispanic trait of machismo could account for Hispanic men taking pride in the amount of alcohol they can ingest without becoming inebriated. The finding may also be a result of the notion that Hispanic Americans seem often to prefer alcohol over drugs. In addition, the socioeconomic pressures faced by Hispanic American men in the United States may be unduly high as a result of job discrimination and social prejudice.

Of particular interest is the observation that Hispanic American women seem to be well protected against alcoholism. This is so not only in comparison to Hispanic American men, but also in comparison to white women. The Catholic religion may be a major factor, because Catholicism perceives alcoholism as a sin. However, other factors would be expected to reinforce the religion element in the case of women, because religion clearly does not exert a powerful protective effect for men. Traditional family influences, mothers' role-modeling, women's general traditional role in the Hispanic culture, and "Marianismo" may indeed also be reinforcing factors (10). "Marianismo" is said to influence Hispanic women in general to behave like the Virgin Mary. It is thought that some Hispanic American women use tranquilizers, such as benzodiazepines, instead of alcohol to deal with the daily pressures of life (11).

It is noteworthy that the peak of alcoholism among Hispanic American men is observed in the 30- to 44-year age group. Hispanic American men in this age bracket would be expected to have already achieved a certain level of education and to have reached good economic positions. However, the connection between income and alcoholism is not clear and does not permit easy explanation.

Among Hispanic American women, the peak of alcoholism is observed primarily in the middle-age (40–59) group. The three factors of high education, income, and acculturation levels have been associated with decreased levels of abstention and/or increased levels of frequent heavy drinking among Hispanic American women (12). It is in this middle-age bracket that these three factors would be expected to be high among Hispanic American women. Furthermore, Hispanic women in that age group would likely be contending with the stress created by the departure of children from the home.

Mexican Americans, as a group, abstain less and drink more than both Puerto Ricans and Cuban Americans. It is interesting to speculate whether Mexican Americans drink more than the other two groups because of their habit of visiting bars and "cantinas" and drinking excessively by themselves (13). Cuban Americans could be more protected against alcoholism as the result of their acculturation style (14). Cuban Americans have primarily used an integrational model of acculturation during their adaptational period in the United States. They have retained, for the most part, their culture of origin, while engaging in considerable interaction with the majority culture. This type of acculturation has been thought to be especially helpful to those confronting acculturative stress, of which alcoholism can be a manifestation (15). For Puerto Ricans, gender and years of residency in the United States are strong predictors for alcoholism (16).

This review has highlighted a complex generational pattern of daily drinking among Mexican American men and women. Among men, daily drinking increases with increasing length of residency in the United States. This pattern is reversed for women. This finding has been suggested to be caused by acculturation levels (17). In this context, the lower the acculturative stress with subsequent generations, the less are the levels of both daily and monthly drinking among Mexican American women. However, such a hypothesis clearly does not explain the male pattern.

Migration patterns demonstrate that recently arrived (1–5 years) Mexican migrant men have higher levels of frequent heavy drinking than Mexican men and United States–born Mexican American men. Also, newly arrived Mexican American men have higher levels of frequent heavy drinking than United States–born Mexican American men. The loss of the network system and the role of acculturative stress (marginalization) among the recently arrived Mexican American men could perhaps be a major influence in this regard (9).

Perhaps the most troubling point with these data is that although Mexican American women in Los Angeles seem relatively well protected against alcoholism, they still show considerable vulnerability to alcohol-related medical problems. It is uncertain whether factors such as tardiness in seeking medical care, lack of health insurance, complications caused by poverty, or other elements account for this state of affairs.

It should be evident that the existing data on drinking patterns among Hispanic Americans permit only hesitant and tenuous conclusions to be drawn. Furthermore, even internal notions about a specific subgroup are inherently problematic. For example, the drinking pattern among Mexican Americans varies as a function of acculturation, therefore weakening the internal consistency of assertions one might make about Mexican American drinking patterns. This alone should argue for efforts to characterize and better understand Hispanic American use and abuse of alcohol.

Formulations and Policy Implications

The findings previously noted and addressed in the discussion section permit elaboration on a series of formulations and/or hypotheses, as well as recommendations directed at public policy considerations. To begin with, we should recognize the relationships that exist between alcoholism and sociodemographic factors. Based on this relationship, we should strongly advocate for efforts directed at improving educational opportunities for Hispanic Americans, particularly for recently arrived Mexican migrants to the United States. Likewise, we must combat discriminatory practices against Hispanic Americans and improve access to jobs and working conditions for them. Furthermore, we should implement, as much as possible, programs directed to diminish the stress experienced by recent migrants from Mexico.

From another perspective, we should also be aware of the vulnerabilities suffered by Hispanic families headed by women. Thus, we should make every effort to attend to the socioeconomic needs of these Hispanic American women and assist them with their day-to-day stresses and tensions.

From a preventive point of view, we should focus on the male and female Hispanic Americans who are very vulnerable to alcoholism. In essence, these are Hispanic American men between ages 30 and 39; Hispanic American women between ages 40 and 49; Mexican American women from first, second, third, and subsequent generations; highly acculturated Hispanic American women; and Hispanic American men who are highly educated and earn high salaries.

We should also dedicate high priority to the investigation of the factors that tend to protect Hispanic American women, in general, against alcoholism and to the factors that produce differences in the rates of alcoholism among Mexican Americans, Puerto Ricans, and Cuban Americans. The study of these factors might lead to the discovery of variables that can be used for the prevention of alcoholism in Mexican Americans in particular, as well as for other Hispanic ethnic minority groups.

It also appears that machismo plays a big role in the excessive consumption of alcohol among Hispanic American men. Thus, we must combat, via education, this negative factor in this population.

Finally, we must make every effort to direct resources to combat alcoholism among recently migrated Mexican Americans. It is this Hispanic subgroup, particularly during their first 5 years of stay in this country, that is more vulnerable to acquiring alcoholism.

References

1. U.S. Bureau of the Census: Current population reports, Series P-20, No 449, 1991
2. Helzer JE, Burnam A, McEvoy LT: Alcohol abuse and dependence, in Psychiatric Disorders in America. Edited by Robins LN, Reigier DA. New York, Free Press, 1991, pp 81–115
3. U.S. Department of Health and Human Services, Public Health Service, Health Resources and Services Administration, Bureau of Health Professions, Division of Disadvantage Assistance: Health Status of Minorities and Low-Income Groups, 3rd Edition. Washington, DC, U.S. Government Printing Office, 1991
4. Burnam MA: Prevalence of alcohol abuse and dependence among Mexican Americans and non-Hispanic whites in the community, in Alcohol Use Among U.S. Ethnic Minorities (Research Monograph No 18). Edited by Spiegler D, Tate D, Aitken S, et al (DHHS Publ No ADM-89-1435). Washington, DC, U.S. Government Printing Office, 1989, pp 163–177
5. National Center for Health Statistics: Drug abuse: ages 12 years to 74 years. Version I: Hispanic Health and Nutrition Examination Survey, 1982–1984. Public Use Data Tape Documentation, Tape No 6543. Washington, DC, U.S. Department of Health and Human Services, Public Health Services, April 1987
6. Alcohol, Drug Abuse and Mental Health Administration: National Clearinghouse for Alcohol and Drug Information, Update. January 1989, p 2
7. Caetano R: Drinking patterns and alcohol problems in a national sample of U.S. Hispanics, in Alcohol Use Among U.S. Ethnic Minorities (Research Monograph No 18). Edited by Spiegler D, Tate D, Aitken S,

et al (DHHS Publ No ADM-89-1435). Washington, DC, U.S. Government Printing Office, 1989, pp 147–162

8. Gilbert MJ: Alcohol-related practices, problems, and norms among Mexican Americans: an overview, in Alcohol Use Among U.S. Ethnic Minorities (Research Monograph No 18). Edited by Spiegler D, Tate D, Aitken S, et al (DHHS Publ No ADM-89-1435). Washington, DC, U.S. Government Printing Office, 1989, pp 115–134
9. Caetano R, Medina Mora ME: Acculturation and drinking among people of Mexican descent in Mexico and the United States. J Stud Alcohol 49(5):462–471, 1988
10. Trotter RT: Mexican-American experience with alcohol, in The American Experience With Alcohol. Edited by Bennett LA, Ames GM. New York, Plenum, 1985, pp 279–296
11. Bryan Page J, Rio J, Sweeney J, et al: Alcohol and adaption to exile in Miami's Cuban population, in The American Experience With Alcohol. Edited by Bennett LA, Ames GM. New York, Plenum, 1985, pp 315–332
12. Gilbert MJ, Cervantes RC: Patterns and practices of alcohol use among Mexican-Americans: a comprehensive review. Hispanic Journal of Behavioral Sciences 8(1):1–60, 1986
13. Gilbert MJ: Mexican-Americans in California: intracultural variations in attitudes and behavior related to alcohol, in The American Experience With Alcohol. Edited by Bennett LA, Ames GM. New York, Plenum, 1985, pp 255–277
14. Ruiz P, Langrod JG: Substance abuse among Hispanic-Americans: current issues and future perspectives, in Substance Abuse: A Comprehensive Textbook. Edited by Lowinson JH, Ruiz P, Millman RB. Baltimore, MD, Williams & Wilkins, 1992, pp 868–874
15. Berry JW, Kim U: Acculturation and mental health, in Health and Cross-Cultural Psychology: Toward Applications. Edited by Dasen P, Berry JW, Sartorious N. London, England, Sage, 1988
16. Fernandez-Pol B, Bluestone H, Morales G, et al: Cultural influences and alcoholism: a study of Puerto Ricans. Alcohol Clin Exp Res 9(5):443–446, 1985
17. Neff JA, Hoppe SK, Perea P: Acculturation and alcohol use: drinking patterns and problems among Anglo and Mexican-American men drinkers. Hispanic Journal of Behavioral Sciences 9(2):151–181, 1987

3

Alcohol and Asian Americans

The prevalence of alcoholism or alcohol abuse/dependence in Asian Americans has been unevenly researched in the literature. Past studies have been lacking in several areas: the uneven use of standardized instruments, poorly defined study groups, and lack of use of diagnostic criteria. One can appreciate the difficulties in studying alcohol consumption in Asian Americans when considering the following factors: research findings in Asian Americans and in Asian citizens in their native countries are often confounding; drinking patterns of Asian Americans in the United States are influenced by the generational status, ethnicity, and social class of the Asian American; and the term *Asian American* implies a homogeneity among Asian ethnic groups that does not exist. Of great concern is that some very populous Asian ethnic groups in the United States, such as Pilipinos and Asian Indians, have not been studied in any meaningful way. Nevertheless, in appraising the current state of research, we will necessarily limit our focus to three particular Asian American groups—Chinese Americans, Japanese Americans, and Korean Americans—selected only because of the dearth of literature and research done on other groups. In this chapter, native Asians will be referred to by the native ethnic group name (e.g., Korean, Chinese), and Asian Americans in the United States will be referred to by the additional term *American* (e.g., Korean American, Chinese American).

It has been generally assumed that alcoholism, or at least heavy drinking, is not a problem for Asian or Asian American communities

(1–3). Many authors assumed this to be the result of sociocultural factors, such as a strong foundation of Confucianist and Taoist beliefs that emphasize moderation. In the late 1970s, research emerged on the physiological effects of alcohol on Asians and Asian Americans, and it was believed that these effects contributed to the presumed limited consumption of alcohol by Asian Americans (4–7). The "flushing response," seen predominantly in Asians and Asian Americans and rarely in whites, is similar to the effects produced by disulfiram, which causes an uncomfortable facial flushing response with warmth, itchiness, and redness, usually beginning in the face and spreading to the trunk and limbs. Concomitant physical symptoms include tachycardia, headache, nausea, dizziness, and drowsiness, which were assumed would make the Asian drinker unable to consume more than modest amounts of alcohol. The sociocultural underpinnings and physiological findings among Asian Americans tended to reinforce the assumption that the total prevalence of heavy alcohol drinking and problem drinking would be extremely low in Asians and Asian Americans.

In our review we examine the reality of this assumption by first presenting the data from the latest small-scale epidemiological studies on alcohol consumption in Asian Americans. Then we discuss the sociocultural and genetic/physiological influences on alcohol consumption for the three major groups under focus (i.e., Chinese, Koreans, and Japanese). We next discuss the implications for future research efforts in alcoholism. Unfortunately, our report will not be able to focus exclusively on alcoholism in Asian Americans because of the dearth of national epidemiological data on Asian Americans and the inconsistent use of structured diagnostic instruments in the studies cited.

There are diverse Asian Pacific ethnic groups in the United States. In 1990, the U.S. Census Bureau reported 7,273,652 Asian and Pacific Islanders living in the United States, or 3.3% of the population. This represents a growth in 10 years of 95% (Table 3–1) (8). The Asian American population varies in terms of ethnicity, education, income, and acculturation, ranging from first- to sixth-generation Chinese Americans to mostly first-generation Vietnamese Americans. Because national sampling strategies have not been developed for Asian Americans as they have for other minority groups, most studies have focused on the major metropolitan areas where there are significant Asian American communities. Therefore, these local data must be interpreted carefully to prevent overgeneralizations to a national sample of Asian Americans.

Table 3–1. Asian Pacific Americans: population by ethnicity: 1980 and 1990

	1980	1990	% Growth
Total Asian Pacific	3,726,440	7,273,662	95
Chinese	806,040	1,645,472	104
Pilipino	774,652	1,406,770	82
Japanese	700,974	847,562	21
Asian Indian	361,531	815,447	125
Korean	354,593	798,849	125
Vietnamese	261,729	614,547	135
Hawaiian	166,814	211,014	26
Samoan	41,948	62,964	50
Guamanian	32,158	49,345	53
Other Asian Pacific	226,001	821,692	264

Source. LEAP Asian Pacific American Public Policy Institute and the UCLA Asian American Studies Center: *The State of Asian Pacific America: A Public Policy Report: Policy Issues to the Year 2020.* Executive Summary, 1992, p. 3.

Rates and Trends of Alcoholism Among Asian Americans

The two best-known studies are those by Chi et al. (9) and by the National Institute on Alcohol Abuse and Alcoholism (NIAAA) (10). The NIAAA study compared Japanese in Japan, Japanese Americans in Hawaii, and Japanese Americans in California with whites in California. The Chi et al. study looked at drinking behavior among three Asian American groups—Chinese Americans, Japanese Americans, and Korean Americans—in Los Angeles.

The NIAAA Study

Table 3–2 presents a main finding of the NIAAA study (10). Comparing the Japanese American men in Santa Clara, California (third or fourth generation), and Hawaii (first generation) with white men, only 30% of Japanese Americans drank three or more times a week, compared with 44% of whites in California and in the United States national sample. Comparing Japanese American women in Santa Clara and Hawaii with white women in Santa Clara and in the United States national sample, only 9% of the Japanese American women drank three or more times

Table 3–2. Overall frequency of drinking among current drinkers by study site and gender

Overall frequency of drinking	Japanese, Japan (*N* = 524)	Japanese ancestry, Oahu, Hawaii (*N* = 199)	Japanese ancestry, Santa Clara, California (*N* = 212)	Whites, Santa Clara, California (*N* = 212)	Whites, U.S. sample[a, b] (*N* = 2,049)
Men (%)					
Three or more times per week	62	32	29	44	44
Once or twice a week	15	24	20	23	22
One to three times a month	16	24	26	20	21
Less than once a month	7	20	26	13	13

Women (%)

Overall frequency of drinking	Japanese, Japan (*N* = 390)	Japanese ancestry, Oahu, Hawaii (*N* = 177)	Japanese ancestry, Santa Clara, California (*N* = 196)	Whites, Santa Clara, California (*N* = 199)	Whites, U.S. sample[a, b] (*N* = 3,078)
Three or more times per week	21	9	9	32	21
Once or twice a week	16	16	16	24	18
One to three times a month	30	23	28	24	32
Less than once a month	33	52	48	20	29

[a]Respondents who reported having a drink in the previous months.
[b]Data are from the 1984 Household Interview Survey by the Alcohol Research Group, Berkeley, California.
Source. Adapted from Kono H, Towle LH, Harford TC: *Alcohol Consumption Patterns and Related Problems in the United States and Japan.* Rockville, MD, National Institute on Alcohol Abuse and Alcoholism, 1991.

a week, compared with 32% of the white women in California and 21% of the white women in the United States national sample. Thus, it appears that Japanese American men and women drink alcohol less frequently than their white counterparts and much less frequently than native Japanese. Despite the fact that the Japanese Americans in the California sample were well acculturated, it still appears that there are protective factors operating against heavy drinking. Indeed, Harford in 1992 (11) demonstrated that family history of alcoholism was lowest in Asian Americans compared with other racial groups using the 1988 National Health Interview Schedule.

The summary report for the NIAAA study concluded with five main points:

1. Most respondents in all four study groups reported being current users of alcoholic beverages.
2. In all study groups a greater proportion of men than women were current drinkers, with native Japanese demonstrating the highest proportion of men to women as current drinkers.
3. More men in Japan than men in any of the United States study sites were classified in the upper categories of alcohol consumption.
4. Among women, more white women drinkers were in the upper categories of amount of drinking, compared with women in Japan or Japanese American women.
5. Among Japanese and Japanese Americans, those who were classified as flushers reported drinking less frequently, drinking smaller amounts of alcohol on the average, and experiencing a lower rate of alcohol problems than nonflushers.

Limitations of the study include the fact that the study was survey based and that there was no attempt at differentiating heavy drinkers from those who might meet criteria for alcohol dependence or alcohol abuse.

The Chi Study

The Chi et al. study (9) compared drinking patterns among Chinese Americans, Korean Americans, and Japanese Americans using the quantity, frequency, and varability criteria from the Cahalan et al. study (12). Among men, the heaviest drinkers (Table 3–3) appear to be, in descending order, Japanese Americans, Korean Americans, and Chinese Americans; infrequent drinking and abstaining were highest in Korean Americans, followed by Japanese Americans and then Chinese Americans. Among

Table 3–3. Alcohol consumption by Asian and white men and women (%)

	Japanese American (N = 235)[a]	Chinese American (N = 218)[a]	Korean American (N = 155)[a]	White American (N = 1,177)[b]
Men				
QFV categories[c]				
Heavy drinkers	28.9	14.2	25.8	21
Light + moderate drinkers	38.3	54.6	28.4	46
Infrequent drinkers + abstainers	32.8	31.2	45.8	33
Women				
QFV categories				
Heavy drinkers	11.7	0.0	0.8	5.0
Light + moderate drinkers	55.0	31.3	17.6	37.0
Infrequent drinkers + abstainers	33.4	68.8	81.6	58.0

Note. QFV = quantity-frequency-variability.
[a]Data from Chi I, Lubben JE, Kitano HH: "Differences in Drinking Behavior Among Three Asian American Groups." *Journal of Studies on Alcohol* 50(1):15–23, 1989.
[b]Cahalan D, Cisin IH, Crossley HM: *American Drinking Practices: A National Study of Drinking Behavior and Attitudes* (Monograph No 6). New Brunswick, NJ, Rutgers Center of Alcohol Studies, 1969.
[c]Abstainers drank less than once a year or not at all. Infrequent drinkers drank at least once a year but less than once a month. Light drinkers drank at least once a month but typically one to two drinks per occasion. Moderate drinkers drank at least once a month but usually no more than three to four drinks per occasion. Heavy drinkers drank nearly every day with five or more drinks per occasion at least once in a while or about once weekly with usually five or more drinks per occasion.

women the pattern was similar, with the highest percentage of heavy drinking found in Japanese American women, followed by Korean Americans and Chinese Americans; infrequent drinking and abstaining were highest in Korean Americans, followed by Chinese Americans and Japanese Americans. It is interesting to note that in Korean American men, the distribution for abstainers and heavy drinkers appears to be impressively bimodal—that is, high numbers of heavy drinkers and high numbers of abstainers. However, interpretation of the Korean American data is limited, as the Korean Americans preferentially sampled were heavily Protestant and reported going to church much more frequently than the Japanese Americans or Chinese Americans in the sample. In contrast, a study by Yamamoto et al. (13) found a high prevalence of alcohol abuse and dependence among elderly Korean American men. In a sample of Korean American senior citizens, 21.6% met criteria for DSM-III-R (14) alcohol abuse and 13.7% met criteria for alcohol dependence. These findings have a very strong concordance with studies done on Koreans in Korea (15, 16). A significant consequence of drinking noted for Korean Americans is that among Asian Americans Koreans appear to have the greatest number of "driving under the influence" charges in Los Angeles

County (17). These data seem to suggest that Korean Americans may be the Asian American group at greatest risk for heavy drinking and problem drinking.

Sociocultural Influences

Studies on Asian American drinking cannot be done without citing comparative statistics with that of the Asian native country. Immigration patterns, as a component of sociocultural factors, likely influence rates and amounts of drinking in Asian Americans (9). As an example, religion is an important aspect of the changing culture among Koreans, as only 25% of native Koreans are Christian, compared with 70% of Korean Americans (18).

As previously stated, it has been popularly accepted by clinicians and laypersons that there is a low rate of alcohol abuse and alcoholism in Asians and Asian Americans. Support for this notion usually is given by the underutilization of hospital and inpatient admissions for alcohol treatment and also the low national morbidity and mortality rates associated with alcohol-induced disease (2, 19). The research literature is replete with both sociocultural and physiological/genetic explanations for this seemingly consistent finding. Sue's excellent review (20) on use and abuse of alcohol by Asian Americans in 1987 gave a clear synopsis of the sociocultural factors that might influence the apparent moderation of drinking in Chinese Americans and Japanese Americans. The two paragraphs that follow summarize Sue's ideas regarding sociocultural influences on drinking.

Historically, sociocultural perspectives with regard to Asian American drinking stressed the importance of cultural values to Chinese, Japanese, and Koreans. In 1970, Hsu (21) argued that the difference in value structures between the American and Chinese ways of life accounts for differences in drinking styles. Hsu believed that the emphasis by Americans on individuality, independence, and assertiveness contributed to increased drinking in Western cultures, because alcohol enhanced these qualities. The Chinese, on the other hand, are more situation centered and "other people centered," with an emphasis on responsibility to others and prescribed behaviors in social situations that make alcohol an unlikely drug for abuse by the Chinese. Among the Chinese, drinking traditionally takes place during meals and is considered to be incidental to eating. The main reason for drinking alcohol is to promote conviviality and improve health. Excessive drinking, drinking alone, and intoxication are strongly discouraged. Especially condemned are aggressive and noisy behaviors when intoxicated (1). Therefore, it is not surprising that few drinking-centered institutions exist for the Chinese in China. This may change as urbanization and free market ideas spread in China, and future studies will be necessary to document any change in drinking patterns.

Traditional Japanese values are similar to those described for the Chinese. The Japanese focus on the value of interdependence, restraint, and group achievement contributes to the controlled and moderated use of alcohol (22, 23). As found in Chinese culture, drinking in Japan is allowed at meals, during ceremonies, and after meetings. However, the rapid change in post–World War II industrialization has clearly influenced alcohol use. The popularity of drinking with friends after work is reported to have increased in relatively recent years, as have the number of bars and nightclubs (24). Nevertheless, in both Chinese and Japanese cultures, there are strong sanctions against drunkenness, especially when associated with aggressive or violent behaviors. Social prohibitions seem to account for the low number of Asian American problem behaviors or crimes related to intoxicated behavior in the United States, Japan, or Hong Kong (1, 3, 25, 26).

Korean Americans are one of the fastest growing immigrant groups in the United States. Most Koreans currently in the United States are first-generation immigrants, and a majority of Korean Americans are affiliated with Protestant churches (18). An excerpt from a book by 59 Korean authors cited by Lubben et al. (26) gives us some insight into the Korean perspective on alcohol consumption in Korea. The general themes are that "drinking is pleasurable, it should be in the company of others, it often involves men accompanied by women, and moderation is desirable" (p. 3). For example, one author wrote that "liquor is creation, friendship, and life," whereas another believed that "life without liquor, women, and money is no life at all" (p. 3). Consistent with the ideas expressed of the importance of alcohol in Korean life, the authors (26) cited Kim (27), who found that 75% of the Korean adult population had used alcohol, and 12% were habitual drinkers, although "habitual" is not defined. Despite these findings, Kim attributed a low rate of serious drinking problems to a social environment that encourages group rather than solitary drinking. Kim also suggested that the Korean public is highly tolerant of alcohol consumption and that Koreans did not view alcoholism as a disease (27). For example, Cho and Faulkner (28) found that Koreans tend to restrict their definition of alcoholism to the physiological consequences of long-term use (cirrhosis, loss of weight, withdrawal symptoms), whereas Americans accept a definition that consists of social and behavioral consequences (e.g., misconduct, problems in role performance). Although the sample size was small and possibly biased (50% refusal rate, and the

Korean sample was older and had more men), these results, if replicated, could have implications for the prevention and treatment of alcoholism for Korean Americans in the United States.

Although the three ethnic groups under study have similar strong sociocultural emphases on family structure and hierarchical relationships and a background of Confucianism that stresses moderation, rapid societal changes since the 1960s parallel alcohol consumption patterns, which are dramatically changing in the native country of these groups. For example, Lee et al. (15) studied the prevalence of psychiatric disorders in Korea by sampling a total of 5,100 subjects using the Diagnostic Interview Schedule; subjects were from Seoul, the urban capital city of South Korea, and rural areas. Applying DSM-III-R (14) criteria for the diagnosis of alcohol abuse/dependence, Lee et al. demonstrated an urban and rural lifetime alcohol abuse/dependence prevalence of about 22%. Comparing this figure to the approximate 15% lifetime prevalence in United States metropolitan areas in the Epidemiologic Catchment Area data (29), one can speculate that alcohol abuse/dependence may be an equal if not greater problem for Koreans than for Americans. In fact, it appears that Korean alcohol intake increased about eightfold between 1960 and 1981. Similarly, Taiwanese Chinese intake increased threefold from 1957 to 1984 (30). One interpretation of these facts posits a causal relationship between continued urbanization and industrialization in Asian societies and an increase in alcohol consumption that may override the "cultural prohibitions" of excessive alcohol use. One concern is that recently arrived immigrant groups may demonstrate or mirror some of these patterns. Whether higher consumption rates in the United States or abroad result in higher comparative rates of undesirable physical and behavioral sequelae of heavy drinking is unknown. However, preliminary evidence does indicate that Japanese men are more likely to exhibit personal problematic symptoms (blackouts and withdrawal), whereas comparative samples of white men in the United States experience more socioproblematic symptoms (e.g., violence, employment, and relationship difficulties) (31). This difference again raises the importance of culture and its effects on the differential perception of problem drinking among Asians and whites. Epidemiological studies to examine these issues are needed but are sorely lacking.

Genetic and Physiological Influences

Wolff (4) observed that many Asians responded to the ingestion of alcohol with a visible flushing reaction that is rarely found in whites. In general, those who flush on drinking generally report lower consumption rates and lower rates of alcohol-related problems than nonflushers. In 1982 Schwitters et al. (32) distinguished "fast flushers" from "slow flushers," with fast flushing defined as one drink or less to evoke flushing and slow flushing defined as two drinks or more to evoke flushing. Schwitters and her colleagues hypothesized and demonstrated that fast flushing would be associated more often with a reduction in drinking than slow flushing. There also appears to be interracial variation; Park et al. in 1984 (33) reported a series of studies done in Hawaii among Koreans and Taiwanese Chinese that showed that significantly more fast flushers were found among Taiwanese Chinese and significantly more slow flushers were found among Koreans (31). Their finding lends support to the hypothesis that typical, or fast, facial flushing seems to be somewhat "protective" against drinking high amounts in Asians.

Facial flushing and other related cardiovascular symptoms are a result of increased blood levels of blood acetaldehyde because of acetaldehyde dehydrogenase type 1 deficiency (ALDH-1) in persons of Asian ancestry (34). Yoshida (35) succinctly explored a model for alcohol sensitivity as related to genetic polymorphisms of alcohol-metabolizing enzymes. Yoshida hypothesized and demonstrated a genomic difference between alcohol flushing subjects and nonflushing subjects, and between alcoholic patients and control subjects in the frequency of the ALDH-1 gene and the atypical Asian type ALDH-2. In his study, virtually all Japanese subjects who exhibited alcohol flushing were heterozygous or homozygous for the atypical ALDH-2 gene, whereas most Japanese patients with alcoholic liver disease were homozygous with the usual ALDH-1 gene. Yoshida concluded that Japanese with genotypes either heterozygous or homozygous for the ALDH-2 gene (the atypical Asian gene) are alcohol sensitive, cannot drink a large amount of alcohol, and do not have a strong alcohol-seeking tendency. Consequently they are at low risk for developing alcohol-related liver diseases. This has been confirmed in Chinese alcoholic patients as well (36, 37).

However, it seems clear that sociocultural factors continue to exert their influence in moderating drinking behavior in nonflushing or heterozygous "flushers." Nakawatase et al. (5) found that Japanese Americans who exhibited the fast flushing response tended to drink less than those who did not flush in a general community sample, but the relationship was weaker in a college student sample. Among the general community sample, there was strong empirical support for the negative relationship between fast flush response and alcohol intake, whereas among college students, there was only weak support.

They found that 50% of the fast flushing group of Japanese American college students was able to have six drinks or more within a 24-hour period. Nakawatase et al. (5) hypothesized that social environmental influences, such as peer pressure, availability of alcoholic beverages, and being away from the strong traditional influences exerted by Asian American parents, could override protection of the ALDH-2 gene (atypical Asian) against alcohol abuse. More recently, Li and Rosenblood (38) impressively demonstrated that cultural norms rather than physical symptoms were highly significant predictors of alcohol consumption patterns for Chinese Canadian and white Canadian university students.

Alcohol-Related Mortality and Morbidity

Table 3–4 illustrates the total death certificate mention rates (total number of times an alcohol-associated diagnosis is mentioned per 100,000 death certificates) for men in the United States in 1980 (39). Except for the report of Korean Americans having the highest rates of driving under the influence (17), it appears that fewer Asian American men experi-

Table 3–4. Death certificate mention rates per 100,000 population, men, United States, 1980

	Racial/ethnic group			
Cause of death (ICD-9-CM code)	**White**	**Chinese**	**Japanese**	**Pilipino**
Alcohol dependence (303)	10.8	1.7	1.2	1.9
Alcoholic liver disease (571.0-3)	9.1	2.7	2.2	3.2
Other liver disease (571.4-9)	20.7	11.3	10.3	8.6
Alcohol abuse (305.0)	2.91	0.7	0.3	1.1
Excess blood level of alcohol (790.3)	0.9	0.2	0.3	0.5
Alcoholic psychosis (291)	0.5	—	—	—
Alcoholic cardiomyopathy (425.5)	0.5	0.2	—	0.3
Alcoholic gastritis (535.3)	0.074	—	—	—
Alcoholic polyneuropathy (357.5)	0.011	—	—	—
Motor vehicle deaths (E810-825)	36.2	10.8	14.6	14.4
Falls (E880-889)	6.5	3.9	5.6	2.9
Fires (E890-899)	2.7	0.5	0.9	0.3
Homicide (E960-969)	10.8	8.8	6.5	6.9
Suicide (E950-959)	19.9	9.1	13.4	5.3

Note. — = no data available.
Source. Adapted from Doufour M, Bertolucci D, Weed J: "Multiple Cause Mortality Data: General Descriptions, Methodological Issues, and Preliminary Findings," in *Alcohol Use Among U.S. Ethnic Minorities* (Research Monograph No 18). Edited by Spiegler D, Tate D, Aitken S, et al (DHHS Publ No ADM-89-1435). Washington, DC, U.S. Government Printing Office, 1989, p. 445.

ence the deleterious consequences of drinking than whites. The numbers for alcohol dependence, alcohol-related liver disease, alcohol abuse, motor vehicle deaths, falls, fires, and suicide are strikingly low for Asian Americans, even when adjusted for the total population of each ethnic group. Caution should be exercised in the interpretation of these data, as rates of heavy drinking appear to be on the rise in Asian countries and the Asian American population in the United States continues to increase. Whether dietary habits, social control exerted by the family, cultural factors, socioeconomic status, or access to health care serve to mitigate the physical and social consequences of heavy drinking in Asian Americans remains unknown.

Summary of the Findings

We can make several conclusions about Asian American drinking:

1. There is a sharp difference between male and female drinking among Asian Americans, with men drinking significantly more than women in all the cultures under study.
2. Japanese Americans and Korean Americans may have the highest proportion of heavy drinkers and Chinese Americans the lowest proportion (9).
3. There may be more Japanese American, Korean American, and Chinese American abstainers (excluding Japanese women) than white abstainers (9).
4. The peak age for drinking for Korean Americans is between 36 and 45 years; for Chinese Americans, between 26 and 35 years; and for Japanese Americans, between 46 and 60 years (9).
5. Asian American heavy drinking is associated with male gender, a tolerant and permissive attitude toward alcohol, having male friends who drink, nonflushing, and lack of embarrassment about flushing (40).
6. Significant morbidity and mortality appear to be lower for Asian American men compared with other racial groups. Chinese men have the lowest number of deaths resulting from alcohol-related cirrhosis and liver disease of any racial group (39).
7. Family history of alcoholism is lowest among Asian Americans compared with other racial groups (11).
8. For Korean Americans, Protestant affiliation may have a protective effect against heavy drinking. For all Asian groups, Confucianist and Taoist beliefs may also be protective.

Discussion

Although there has been a widespread belief that Asians and Asian Americans as a group do not drink heavily, this has been shown not to be so (9, 10, 13). There are significant differences in drinking among the various Asian ethnic groups, and it appears that Chinese Americans drink much less than Japanese Americans and Korean Americans. As in their ancestral countries, Asian American men drink more heavily than women, and Asian women drink significantly less often than women in the United States and Europe (12, 13, 41, 42).

For Korean Americans, a strong Protestant religious faith may be highly protective. For example, Koreans tended to drink as heavily as Japanese in their home countries, but in the United States it appears that Protestant Korean Americans drink slightly less than Japanese Americans (15, 16). Protestant religion plays an important role in the United States for Korean Americans, as 70% of them become Protestant, compared with only 25% of the Koreans in Korea (18). This strong affiliation with Protestant Korean churches fosters a subcultural feeling of disapproval for heavy use of alcohol, as has been true among the most fundamentalist Protestant groups in the United States. Therefore, when assessing Korean American drinking, one must always ask about adherence to Protestant religious faith.

There are also genetic and physiological influences on drinking among Asian Americans (4, 35). These influences are not absolute, as can be shown by the data for Japanese Americans and Korean Americans who both have a significant proportion of flushers and yet seem to also have a high proportion of heavy drinkers (9). Whether Chinese Americans have a higher proportion of "fast flushers" compared with Japanese Americans and Korean Americans as an explanation for the significant differences among these three groups is intriguing but will require further study.

By current statistical measures, Asian Americans in the United States seem to have disproportionately fewer alcohol-related problems than other minority groups. It has been assumed that this is a result of some sociocultural protective factors, as well as genetic and physiological protective factors. It will be interesting over the next decade to continue to examine alcohol consumption research in China, Korea, and the United States as the Asian countries rapidly industrialize. Conventional wisdom suggests that one might expect higher levels of alcohol consumption and consequences of drinking, but this may not be necessarily so if traditional sociocultural factors exert their influence by successfully moderating the more deleterious public health consequences of drinking. In addition, continued acculturative processes in the United States for Asian Americans also provide fertile areas of study. One can hypothesize that as minority groups in general, and Asian Americans in particular, become more acculturated, they will begin to emulate the drinking patterns of the larger majority. However, thus far this appears not to be the case for third- and fourth-generation Japanese Americans in Hawaii or Santa Clara, California, as evidenced by the smaller numbers of heavy drinkers compared with whites. This "protection" among Japanese Americans, which is not seen among Japanese, has been explained as the impact of "enculturation" in the Japanese (43). Kitano et al. (43) believe that post–World War II Japanese were influenced by the American occupation, rapid urbanization and industrialization, and a questioning of traditional values (enculturation), whereas Japanese Americans instead felt the gradual effects of residing in the United States (acculturation). Therefore, it is possible that Japanese Americans drink less because they still retain more pre-World War II drinking values than Japanese in Japan.

Given the ongoing debate between those who ardently believe that alcohol abuse/dependence has a genetic basis and those who believe that environmental/social factors have the greatest importance, it is unfortunate that more epidemiological, diagnostic, and treatment research has not been done on Asian Americans, especially because the study of alcohol abuse/dependence in Asian Americans clearly involves sociocultural and genetic influences. However, current research is variably limited by the lack of national sampling strategies for Asian Americans, the tremendous heterogeneity among Asian American groups, little dissemination of cross-culturally valid diagnostic instruments and few bilingual/bicultural treatment models. More refined studies on the nature of alcoholism (and alcoholism treatment) in Asians and Asian Americans may point the way toward a more reasoned allocation of resources in overall national research efforts to combat alcoholism. In addition, there is much to gain by encouraging pilot studies on the little-known drinking patterns of increasingly large Asian ethnic groups such as Pilipinos and Asian Indians. A more clear description of the prevalence of alcohol dependence in these groups would help Asian American communities to target scarce resources toward prevention in groups with high morbidity from alcoholism. Whatever the outcome, we believe that the continued elucidation of the complex interplay between sociocultural and genetic/physiological influences on drinking behavior in Asian Americans will shed new light and raise questions relevant to all alcohol researchers.

References

1. Chu G: Drinking patterns and attitudes of roominghouse Chinese in San Francisco. Q J Stud Alcohol 6 (suppl):58–68, 1972
2. Singer K: Drinking patterns and alcoholism in the Chinese. Br J Addict 67:3–14, 1972
3. Singer K: The choice of intoxicants among the Chinese. Br J Addict 69:257–268, 1974
4. Wolff P: Ethnic differences in alcohol sensitivity. Science 175:449–450, 1972
5. Nakawatase T, Yamamoto J, Sasao T: The association between fast flushing response and alcohol use among Japanese Americans. J Stud Alcohol 54:48–53, 1993
6. Agarwal DP, Harada S, Goedde HW: Racial differences in biological sensitivity to ethanol: the role of alcohol dehydrogenase and aldehyde dehydrogenase isozymes. Alcohol Clin Exp Res 5:12–16, 1981
7. Higuchi S, Parrish K, Dufour M, et al: The relationship between three subtypes of the flushing response and DSM-III alcohol abuse in Japanese. J Stud Alcohol 53:553–560, 1991
8. LEAP Asian Pacific American Public Policy Institute and the UCLA Asian American Studies Center: The State of Asian Pacific America: A Public Policy Report: Policy Issues to the Year 2020. Executive Summary, 1992, p. 3 (unpublished document)
9. Chi I, Lubben JE, Kitano HH: Differences in drinking behavior among three Asian American groups. J Stud Alcohol 50(1):15–23, 1989
10. National Institute on Alcohol Abuse and Alcoholism, Rockville, Maryland, USA and National Institute on Alcoholism, Kurihama National Hospital, Yokosuka, Kanagawa, Japan: Alcohol Consumption Patterns and Related Problems in the United States and Japan: Summary Report of a Joint United States Japan Alcohol Epidemiological Project. Washington, DC, U.S. Government Printing Office, September 1991
11. Harford T: Family history of alcoholism in the United States: prevalence and demographic characteristics. Br J Addict 87:931–935, 1992
12. Cahalan D, Cisin IH, Crossley HM: American Drinking Practices: A National Study of Drinking Behavior and Attitudes (Monograph No 6). New Brunswick, NJ, Rutgers Center of Alcohol Studies, 1969
13. Yamamoto J, Rhee S, Chang DS: Psychiatric disorder among elderly Koreans in the United States. Community Ment Health J 30(1):17–27, 1994

14. American Psychiatric Association: Diagnostic and Statistical Manual of Mental Disorders, 3rd Edition, Revised. Washington, DC, American Psychiatric Assocation, 1987
15. Lee CK, Kwak YS, Yamamoto J, et al: Psychiatric epidemiology in Korea, part II: urban and rural differences. J Nerv Ment Dis 178(4):247–252, 1990
16. Lee CK, Kwak YS, Yamamoto J, et al: Psychiatric epidemiology in Korea, part I: gender and age differences in Seoul. J Nerv Ment Dis 178(4):242–246, 1990
17. Special Service for Groups: Asian Pacific Alcohol Peer Consultation Training Project: Needs Assessment. Los Angeles, CA, 1991 (unpublished document)
18. Hurh WM, Kim KC: Korean Immigrants in America. Cranbury, NJ, Associated University Presses, 1984
19. Izuno T, Miyakawa M, Tsunoda T, et al: Alcohol-related problems encountered by Japanese, Caucasian, and Japanese Americans. Int J Addict 27(12):1389–1400, 1992
20. Sue D: Use and abuse of alcohol by Asian Americans. J Psychoactive Drugs 19(1):57–66, 1987
21. Hsu FLK: Americans and Chinese. New York, Doubleday, 1970
22. Yamamoto J, Kubota M: The Japanese American family, in The Psychosocial Development of Minority Group Children. Edited by Powell GL. New York, Brunner/Mazel, 1983
23. Lebra TS: Japanese Patterns of Behavior. Honolulu, University of Hawaii Press, 1976
24. Kitano HHL, Hatanaka H, Yeung WT, et al: Japanese American drinking patterns, in The American Experience With Alcohol. Edited by Bennett LA, Ames GA. New York, Plenum, 1985
25. Wang RP: A study of alcoholism in Chinatown. Int J Soc Psychiatry 14:260–267, 1966
26. Lubben J, Chi I, Kitano HHL: The relative influence of selected social factors on Korean drinking behavior in Los Angeles. Adv Alcohol Subst Abuse 8(1):1–17, 1989
27. Kim KI: Culture and mental disorder in Korea. Plenary session: culture and psyche in Korea, in Proceedings of the Second Pacific Congress of Psychiatry, May 23–25, 1980. Seoul, Korea, Korean Neuropsychiatric Association, 1980, pp 17–23
28. Cho YI, Faulkner WR: Conceptions of alcoholism among Koreans and Americans. Int J Addict 28(8):681–694, 1993
29. Robins LN, Regier DA (eds): Psychiatric Disorders in America: The Epidemiologic Catchment Area Study. New York, Free Press, 1991, pp 84–86

30. Yamamoto J, Yeh EK, Lee CK, et al: Alcohol abuse among Koreans and Taiwanese, in Cultural Influences and Drinking Patterns: A Focus on Hispanic and Japanese Populations (Research Monograph No 19). Edited by Towle LH, Harford TC (DHHS Publ No ADM-88-1563). Washington, DC, U.S. Government Printing Office, 1988, pp 135–175
31. Izuno, T, Miyakawa M, Tsunoda T, et al: Alcohol related problems encountered by Japanese, Caucasians, and Japanese Americans. Int J Addict 27(12):1389–1400, 1992
32. Schwitters SY, Johnson RC, McGlearn GE, et al: Alcohol use and the flushing response in different racial-ethnic groups. J Stud Alcohol 43:1259–1262, 1982
33. Park JY, Huang YH, Nagoshi CT, et al: The flushing response to alcohol use among Koreans and Taiwanese. J Stud Alcohol 45: 481–485, 1984
34. Mizoi Y, Tatsuno Y, Adachi J, et al: Alcohol sensitivity related to polymorphism of alcohol metabolizing enzyme in Japanese. Pharmacol Biochem Behav 18 (suppl 1):127–133, 1983
35. Yoshida A: Genetic polymorphism of alcohol metabolizing enzymes related to alcohol sensitivity and alcoholic diseases, in Psychopharmacology and Psychobiology of Ethnicity. Edited by Lin KM, Poland R, Nakasaki G. Washington, DC, American Psychiatric Press, 1993, pp 169–183
36. Harada S: Genetic polymorphism of aldehyde dehydrogenase and its physiological significance to alcohol metabolism. Prog Clin Biol Res 344:289–291, 1990
37. Thomasson HR, Edenberg HJ, Crabb DW, et al: Alcohol and aldehyde dehydrogenase genotypes and alcoholism in Chinese men. Am J Hum Genet 48:677–681, 1991
38. Li HZ, Rosenblood L: Exploring factors influencing alcohol consumption patterns among Chinese and Caucasian. J Stud Alcohol 55:427–433, 1994
39. Dufour M, Bertolucci D, Weed J: Multiple cause mortality data: general descriptions, methodological issues, and preliminary findings, in Alcohol Use Among U.S. Ethnic Minorities (Research Monograph No 18). Edited by Spiegler D, Tate D, Aitken S, et al (DHHS Publ No ADM-89-1435). Washington, DC, U.S. Government Printing Office, 1989, p 445
40. Parrish KM, Higuchi S, Stinson FS, et al: Genetic or cultural determinants of drinking: a study of embarrassment at facial flushing among Japanese and Japanese Americans. J Subst Abuse 2(4): 439–447, 1990

41. Hwu HG, Yeh EK, Chang LY: Prevalence of psychiatric disorders in Taiwan defined by the Chinese Diagnostic Interview Schedule. Acta Psychiatr Scand 79:136–147, 1989
42. Helzer JE, Canino GJ, Yeh EK, et al: Alcoholism in North America and Asia. Arch Gen Psychiatry 47:313–319, 1990
43. Kitano HHL, Chi I, Rhee S, et al: Norms and alcohol consumption: Japanese in Japan, Hawaii and California. J Stud Alcohol 53:33–39, 1992

4

Alcohol and Native Americans

Defining the precise variables that characterize and define each ethnic group may be more elusive and arbitrary than is apparent in this monograph thus far. Most large-scale epidemiological studies, such as the Epidemiologic Catchment Area (ECA) study as well as local institutional or regional studies, have relied on comparisons between groups defined according to United States historical-political categories rather than according to operationally defined ethnic variables. Most "majority" as well as "minority" Americans more or less agree that they are able to categorize themselves and others as white (Caucasian), black (African American), Asian American, Hispanic American, or Native American. Such identifications are often heartfelt and passionately proclaimed and defended. Closer examination, however, reveals that the variables used to define these categories are neither exclusive nor comparable in the same dimensions, thus exposing a true "apples-and-oranges" dilemma for the cultural scientist. Estimates of skin color define "blacks" and "whites." Spanish as "native language" spoken by self or ancestors defines "Hispanics." Continent of origin defines "Asian Americans." Arrival in America during the past 400 years presumably differentiates Asian Americans from "Native Americans," whose ancestors arrived from Asia in several different migrating periods some thousands of years ago. Some Native American groups and individuals therefore physically resemble some Asian Americans. Some Native American groups use Spanish as their native language and may be categorized as Hispanic. In the southeastern United States, some Native American groups use French as their mother tongue and have ancestors that were brought from Africa as slaves. They may be variously categorized as Creoles, Indians, or blacks depending on the situation and purpose of the classification. Some white-appearing individuals may classify themselves as Native American based on identifications with a grandparent or more distant ancestor. Boundaries precisely differentiating Native Americans from the other groups considered in this monograph are often therefore lacking.

Among those groups in which the above ambiguities are minimal, there are still few genetic, linguistic, or cultural features that would distinguish them as a single ethnic entity for purposes of epidemiological comparisons with the other "major" ethnic minority groups in the United States. In fact, there is tremendous variation and diversity among the many groups that are officially and unofficially considered Native American. There are 309 tribal groups currently defined and an additional 200 "native entities" in Alaska. Linguistic and cultural differences are significant, with more than 200 distinct languages (1), probably stemming from three major language groups, each representing a geohistorical period characterized by major migration of different people from northern Asia.

Native Americans and Alaska Natives number about 1.5 million, or less than 1% of the total United States population of 250 million. The most concentrated numbers of Native Americans are on reservations and in the pueblos of the Southwest. Whereas most Alaska Natives live in villages and towns geographically distant and isolated from the cities, 52% of Native Americans in the lower 48 states currently live in urban areas. Many of these are transient, moving from tribal village or reservation to the city and back, depending on job, family, education, health, and recreational circumstances. Obtaining an adequately representative sample for epidemiological studies of alcoholism in such a mobile, widely dispersed, and heterogeneous population has not yet been feasible. The data that do exist regarding alcohol use and abuse in this widely dispersed heterogeneous group are therefore not directly comparable with the national sampling data presented for black, Hispanic, and Asian American groups in previous chapters.

The notion that Native Americans are constitutionally more vulnerable to becoming dependent on alcohol has become known as the "firewater myth." In fact, as we discuss later, many tribes actually abstain or drink less and have lower rates of problems with alcohol than the United States population at large. In addition, several authorities have pointed out that the white colonists actually provided models of drinking as an expression of power and prestige for Indians to emulate throughout the centuries of their Western expansion and usurpation of Native American lands.

On the other hand, notions of power being associated with altered states of consciousness and trance were syncretic ideas in some ways harmonious with some Native American practices that associated personal spiritual power with the trance state. For example, the tradition of the guardian spirit quest among the Sioux Indians, peyotism in the Native American Church among the Navaho and other Southwest Indian groups, and soul voyages of the shaman in numerous Native American tribes place value on the controlled altered state of consciousness as a "religious" experience. Although most Native Americans would consider using alcohol to be antithetical and an abomination to their religious beliefs, many studies (2–5) indicate that one goal of drinking is to become quickly entranced. In the altered state of consciousness produced by intoxication, the individual can temporarily experience a euphoria that brings with it a sense of power and self-assertion, not unlike the power sought in a shamanistic trance.

Rates and Trends

Attitudes toward drinking alcohol vary considerably from tribe to tribe. For example, the Navaho accept social drinking as normative and use alcohol off the reservation for recreational and celebratory purposes. On the other hand, the Hopi, who live in the Southwest, view drinking alcohol as irresponsible and a threat to their religious value of cosmic harmony (2). This is not meant to imply that there is necessarily any unanimity within tribes regarding adherence to these norms and values. For example, 48% of Navajo actually abstain totally from alcohol, compared with 16%–20% abstinence found among various other groups. The same degree of variation is seen between and within tribes when one examines the heavy use of alcohol. For example, among Indians of the Southwest tribes, including the Navaho, only 14% are considered heavy drinkers (2) in contrast to 26%–42% among the various other groups compared above (5–8).

Since the 1960s, the number of Native Americans who have migrated from rural tribal areas to cities has increased dramatically. In 1960 only 18% of Native Americans lived in cities. By 1990, 52% of the Native American population were living in urban areas. Several studies indicate that urban Native Americans drink more heavily than those who remain in rural areas. For example, among one group living in an eastern city, 33% were found to be heavy drinkers, compared with 19% of a second group from the same tribe who lived in a nearby rural county (9).

Among Native Americans living in Los Angeles, 16% have been found to drink heavily, compared with 5.8% of California Indians living in rural areas (10).

Treatment Utilization

One measure of alcohol problems in a population is the utilization of hospitals for treatment of alcoholism and related illnesses. Table 4–1 compares hospital utilization rates for the white majority and for several ethnic minority groups. The data show that overall, men ages 25–44 and nonwhites are overrepresented in inpatient treatment settings for alcohol and substance abuse. In this table, data for Native Americans and Asian Americans have been combined because of their small numbers; together they represent only 3% of the total population in the United States treated for alcohol abuse/dependency. Despite popular perceptions, the data illustrate that by national standards, alcoholism among Native Americans is a minuscule burden on the country's medical services compared with other groups. However, hospital and clinic utilization rates by Native Americans may be artificially low because of their lack of access to medical care, including hospitals, as well as the cultural incongruity of hospital treatment facilities and personnel. Nevertheless, in Alaska, one study found that Alaska Natives represented 65% of the alcohol-treatment population, despite making up only 17% of the general population (11). Based on treatment utilization and morbidity statistics, the National Health Service estimates that overall, 40% of Native Americans are problem heavy drinkers, compared with only 14% of whites (12).

Table 4–1. Patients in alcohol and drug treatment, United States, 1990

	Treatment population (%)	General population (%)
Men	72	50
White	62	80
Black	21	12
Hispanic	14	6
Native American and Asian American	3	< 1 + 2
Ages 25–44	> 50	

Male-Female Drinking Patterns

On a national basis, Native American women represent less than one-fourth of treated problem drinkers (12). However, studies of gender differences in susceptibility to problem drinking in several different tribes have been contradictory. Reports indicate that heavy alcohol use in women decreases after the young adult years (ages 18–25), and women are more likely than men to maintain abstinence (8, 13). However, studies of certain Native American groups in the Midwest and in Alaska have revealed high rates of alcohol problems in women (10, 14).

Some Native American women seem to be especially at risk for cirrhosis of the liver. Cirrhosis of the liver has been used as an indirect indicator of alcoholism, although other factors such as nutritional deficiencies and hepatitis commonly found in Native American groups confound this conclusion. Nevertheless, rates of cirrhosis are significantly higher for Native American women compared with rates for white women. In 1980, for example, cirrhotic death rates in Native American women were found to be 16 per 100,000, compared with 3.4 per 100,000 for the white female population of the United States (15).

The risk of developing alcoholic cirrhosis is based not only on constitutional and nutritional factors, but also on styles of drinking, which also vary considerably from tribe to tribe. For example, the recreation "binge" style of drinking seen among the Navaho is accompanied by lower cirrhotic rates and low rates of fetal alcohol syndrome (1.3 per 100,000). In contrast, among the Plains tribes, where those who drink are inclined more toward daily consumption patterns, rates of cirrhosis and fetal alcohol syndrome (10.3 per 100,000) are much higher (16, 17).

In 1987 the treatment rate among Native Americans for liver cirrhosis was found to be 64 per 100,000, in contrast to 19 per 100,000 for the general United States population. Alcoholism was considered to be the prime causal factor in about 85% of cases of cirrhosis among Native Americans. The age-adjusted mortality rate for liver cirrhosis in Native American men in 1980 was 33 per 100,000, in contrast to the United States population cirrhotic death rate of 13.2 per 100,000.

As in the cases of cirrhosis of the liver and fetal alcohol syndrome, rates of death resulting directly from alcohol dependence, psychosis, and liver failure vary dramatically from one tribe to another. Among the Creek and Cherokee, alcohol-related mortality rates are comparatively low (6 per 100,000), whereas among other groups, rates are phenomenally high (92–239 per 100,000) (18, 19). The overall mortality rates from these causes are still 4.5 times higher among Native Americans (38 per 100,000) than among the general United States population (7.8 per 100,000) (Figure 4–1) (20).

Age-Related Patterns of Alcohol Use and Abuse

Several large-scale surveys of alcohol and drug use have been conducted in Native American middle and high school students. Oetting and Beauvais (21) surveyed five southwest Native American groups, and Blum et al. (22) studied eight Native American health service areas, including 37 separate units. Both studies compared alcohol use patterns among Native American youth with those found in whites and other ethnic minority populations. Their findings were similar, showing that by the 12th grade, most students had tried alcohol at least once (whites, 79%; Native Americans, 89%). Only 12% of Native Americans and 16% of whites, however, continued to drink on a daily or weekly basis. About 60% of Native American youth did not drink at all. Of those who did use alcohol, 20% were infrequent users, but heavy recreational drinking was the norm among another 20%. Forty-six percent of Native American youths who drank said that they did so to get drunk, in contrast to 23% of white drinkers of the same age. Native American youth who

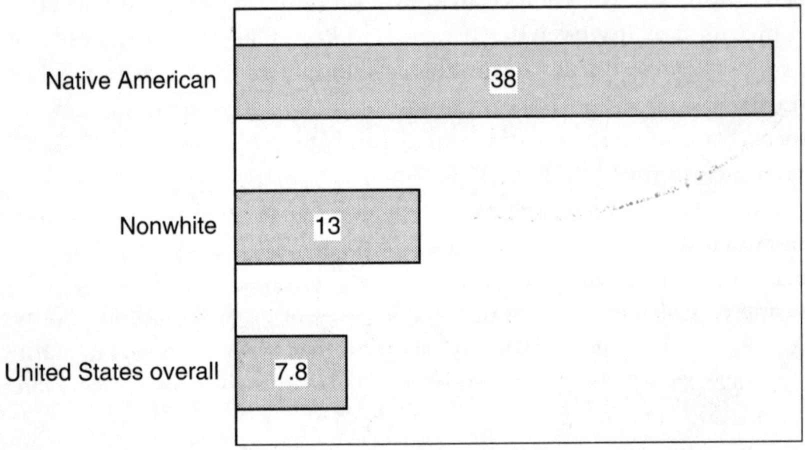

Figure 4–1. American Indian alcohol related death rates (dependence/psychosis/alcoholic cirrhosis). Rates are per 100,000 people.
Source. Mason R, Mail P, Palmer I, et al: *Briefing Book for the Alcohol Program Review*. Albuquerque, NM, Program Branch, Indian Health Service, 1985.

drank also had more severe social problems than those who did not. They had 2.5 times more accidents, twice the frequency of school problems, three times more suicide attempts, and three times more family problems, including incidence of abuse, than nonusers. In contrast with the majority population, Native American youths experienced alcohol-related arrest rates that were 10 times higher than those of comparably aged whites and a suicide rate that was more than twice that for whites (26.3 vs. 12.4 per 100,000) (21).

Many of the trends found in youths and associated with alcohol problems continue into adulthood. Native Americans have 2.3 times the suicide rate of the white population, 2.8 times the homicide rate, and three times the accidental death rate, with automobile accident death rates 5.5 times higher than those of whites. About 80% of deaths reported in these categories for Native Americans are associated with alcohol abuse (Table 4–2) (15).

Summary of the Findings

Taking into consideration the caveats noted previously regarding tribal variations in culture, language, geography, customs, and drinking patterns, several generalizations regarding Native American alcohol use do emerge from the data presented:

1. Native American communities overall include a substantial proportion of individuals who abstain from alcohol.
2. There are few moderate drinkers.
3. Of those who do drink, most drink heavily, which in the context of poverty, poor general health, and frequently hazardous environmental conditions results in high rates of alcohol-related morbidity and mortality.

Table 4–2. Alcohol-related problems

Native Americans compared with majority population have

- 3x Alcohol-related illnesses
- 4.2x Alcohol-related mortality rates
- 3x Accidental death rate (an estimated three-fourths are alcohol related)
- 2.3x Suicide rate (an estimated 80% are alcohol related)
- 2.8x Homicide rate (an estimated 90% are alcohol related)

4. Drinking is heaviest in men ages 25–44, and a pattern of heavy, hazardous drinking is established during high school years.
5. Women who drink have a high risk for alcohol-related morbidity in themselves and their offspring.
6. The rate of consumption decreases, the number of drinkers declines, and the percentage of abstainers increases during middle age, leaving fewer older individuals with alcohol problems (23–25).

Discussion

The consequences of alcohol use in terms of sickness, physical and emotional suffering, and death in Native American groups where heavy drinking is prevalent have been tragic. In spite of federal and local indigenous efforts to control excessive alcohol use in these groups, problems continue. As a result, the image of the "drunken Indian" continues to be unfairly perpetuated in national lore, undermining further efforts of Native American communities and individuals to find acceptance, pride, and achievement in the national context.

Research findings have linked alcohol abuse in teenagers to abuse by parents and other caretakers. Child abuse may be associated with poverty. Unemployment and underemployment are high among Native Americans. The average size of the Native American family is large (four to five children). Parental age is often relatively young. Those individuals who were abused in childhood themselves become child abusers in later life, creating a self-perpetuating cycle of alcohol use and self-defeating behaviors recurring through generations. Harford (26) reported that a random sample of Native Americans acknowledged a positive family history of alcoholism at rates significantly higher than in other ethnic minority groups in the United States, with 46% of Native American men and 63% of Native American women reporting such family histories.

In contrast, individuals who can identify with a traditional Native American family and cultural ways and/or who have learned to believe that they and their families can be successful in the dominant society seem to be at less risk for problems associated with drugs and alcohol. Oetting and Beauvais (21) found that high school students who identified with living and succeeding in the "Native American way" had a lower risk for morbidity associated with alcohol than those who did not endorse these items. Native American students who identified themselves with Native American ways and with success in the "white-American way" were most likely to do well in school, have higher self-esteem, and avoid heavy alcohol use. Oetting and Beauvais (21) have argued that biculturality (i.e., having positive attitudes toward and involvement in both cultures) is the best protection against morbidity associated with alcohol. This is supported by another study of a Native American adult population in Alaska, where Klausner and Foulks (14) found that those individuals who were church attenders, held salaried jobs, and had bicultural identifications were significantly less likely to manifest problems with drinking alcohol.

The relationship between alcohol use and church membership and attendance and/or traditional ceremonial participation is a subject worthy of further research. In a study of a large sample from Plains, Plateau, and Pueblo groups, Manson et al. (27) reported that comparing the 63% of the total sample who were church members with the remainder who were not revealed no significant difference in abuse (24% vs. 15%) or dependency on alcohol (31% vs. 30%). Comparing the 45% who participated in traditional ceremonials with those who did not also revealed no significant differences (20% vs. 24% abused alcohol and 33% vs. 22%, respectively, were dependent). However, the authors did not report on the alcohol use of those who were church members and participated in traditional ceremonials, which may have provided further insights into the hypothetical relationship between bicultural adaptation as a preventive factor for alcohol-related disorders. Such a comparison may have provided an indication of the degree to which bicultural identifications inoculate against excessive use of alcohol and associated problems. Based on a review of the literature on biculturalism, LaFromboise et al. (28) identified sets of skills related to bicultural competence; these include the ability to form stable social networks in both cultures and to utilize these external support systems, knowledge of beliefs and values of both cultures, positive attitudes toward both groups, communication competency, cross-cultural social skills, and confidence that one can live within two groups without compromising one's sense of cultural identity.

Treatment Research Implications

A related question regards the availability and utilization of those healing paradigms offered not only by Western biomedicine but by non-Western spiritual and religious institutions as well. Can a combination of these be used therapeutically to alleviate alcohol problems in Native Americans? Such approaches may be complicated by the great variation in traditional healing practices between tribes. On the other hand, a "Pan–Native American" perspective has brought a widespread acceptance of the "sweat lodge" and other traditional ceremonies that require abstinence from alcohol in preparation for a sought-after spiritual experience. Basic to many of these traditional ceremonial approaches to healing is the notion that alcohol is an impurity introduced by a foreign society that interferes with obtaining a natural harmonious balance between self, society, and nature.

Jilek (29) has provided an overview of the variety of Native American ceremonial practices and religious observances that are currently being utilized as a response to alcohol abuse and the psychosocial problems currently experienced by many groups. His review includes detailed discussion of the "inupiaq ilitqsat" (Eskimo spirit movement), the "sun dance," the "winter spirit dance," the Plains Indians' "gourd dance," the Native American Church "peyote cult," the "gaiwiio," and "Amerind-AA" groups.

Ethnic revitalization movements such as those currently utilized by Native Americans may provide a model for other oppressed minority groups to follow in developing social treatments and preventive strategies to address the problems of alcohol abuse and dependency, as well as abuse and dependency involving other substances. We believe that outcome studies will demonstrate that such ethnic revitalization resources not only will prove effective for substance disorders, but also will create the solidarity and self-determination required to discover solutions to most of their psychosocial problems in the most culturally sensitive way.

References

1. French L: Indians and Criminal Justice. Totowa, NJ, Allanheld, Osmun & Company, 1982
2. Levy JE, Kunitz S: Indian Drinking: Navaho Practices and Anglo-American Theories. New York, Wiley, 1974
3. Foulks D: The transformations of Arctic hysteria, in Culture-Bound Syndromes. Edited by Simons R, Hughes C. Boston, MA, D Reidel, 1985, pp 307–325
4. Young TJ: Substance use and abuse among Native Americans. Clin Psychol Rev 8:125–138, 1988
5. Jessor R, Graves T, Hanson R, et al: Society, Personality, and Deviant Behavior: A Study of a Tri-Ethnic Community. New York, Holt, Reinhart & Winston, 1969
6. Longclaws L, Barnes G, Grieve L, et al: Alcohol and drug use among the Brokenhead Ojibwa. J Stud Alcohol 41:21–36, 1980

7. May P: Substance abuse and American-Indians. Int J Addict 17(7):1185–1209, 1982
8. May P: Alcohol abuse and alcoholism among American Indians: an overview, in Alcoholism in Minority Populations. Edited by Watts T, Roosevelt W. Springfield, IL, Charles C Thomas, 1989, pp 95–119
9. Beltrame T, McQueen D: Urban and rural Indian drinking patterns: the special case of the Lumbee. Int J Addict 14(4):533–548, 1979
10. Weibel-Orlando J, Weisner T, Long J: Urban and rural Indian drinking patterns: implications for intervention and policy development. Subst Alcohol Actions Misuse 5:45–57, 1984
11. Mala T: Status of mental health of Alaska Natives. Alaska Med 21: 1–3, 1979
12. Lewis R: Alcoholism and the Native Americans—a review, in Alcohol and Health Monograph No 4 (National Institute on Alcohol Abuse and Alcoholism, Special Publication issues, DHHS Publ No ADM-82-1193). Washington, DC, U.S. Government Printing Office, 1982
13. Heath D: Alcohol use among North American Indians: a cross-cultural survey of patterns and problems, in Research Advances in Alcohol and Drug Problems No 7. Edited by Smart R, Glaser F, Israel Y, et al. New York, Plenum, 1983, pp 341–396
14. Klausner S, Foulks E: Eskimo Capitalists: Oil, Politics, and Alcohol. Totowa, NJ, Allanheld, Osmun & Company, 1982
15. Dufour M, Bertolucci D, Weed J: Multiple cause mortality data: general descriptions, methodological issues, and preliminary findings, in Alcohol Use Among U.S. Ethnic Minorities (Research Monograph No 18). Edited by Spiegler D, Tate D, Aitken S, et al (DHHS Publ No ADM-89-1435). Washington, DC, U.S. Government Printing Office, 1989, pp 439–450
16. May P, Hymbaugh K, Aase J, et al: Epidemiology of fetal-alcohol syndrome among American Indians of the Southwest. Soc Biol 30:374–387, 1983
17. Weibel-Orlando J: IHS, Alcohol Abuse and Future Research Directions: Review of the Indian Health Service Alcoholism Program. Denver, CO, U.S. Government Printing Office, 1985
18. Cohen S: Alcohol and the Indian. Drug Abuse and Alcoholism Newsletter 11(4):1, 1982
19. Berman T: Suicide among the Shoshone-Paiute on the Duck Valley Reservation. Owyee, NV, Shoshone Paiute Tribe, 1970 (unpublished manuscript)

20. Mason R, Mail P, Palmer I, et al: Briefing Book for the Alcohol Program Review. Albuquerque, NM, Program Branch, Indian Health Service, 1985
21. Oetting E, Beauvais F: Epidemiology and correlates of alcohol use among Indian adolescents living on reservations, in Alcohol Use Among U.S. Ethnic Minorities (Research Monograph No 18). Edited by Spiegler D, Tate D, Aitken S, et al (DHHS Publ No ADM-89-1435). Washington, DC, U.S. Government Printing Office, 1989, pp 239–267
22. Blum R, Harmon B, Harris L, et al: American Indian-Alaska Native youth health. JAMA 267:1637–1644, 1992
23. Lex B: Alcohol problems in special populations, in The Diagnosis and Treatment of Alcoholism, 2nd Edition. Edited by Mendelson J, Mello N. New York, McGraw-Hill, 1985, pp 89–187
24. Leland JH: Native American alcohol use: a review of the literature, in Tulapai to Tokay. Edited by Mail P, McDonald D. New Haven, CT, HRAF Press, 1980, pp 1–56
25. Lemert EM: Drinking among American Indians, in Alcohol, Science, and Society Revisited. Edited by Gomberg E, White H, Carpenter J. Ann Arbor, University of Michigan Press, 1982, pp 80–95
26. Harford TC: Family history of alcoholism in the United States: prevalence and demographic characteristics. Br J Addict 87:931–935, 1992
27. Manson S, Shore J, Baron A, et al: Alcohol abuse and dependency among American Indians, in Alcoholism in North America, Europe and Asia. Edited by Holzer J, Canino G. New York, Oxford University Press, 1992
28. LaFromboise T, Coleman H, Gerton J: Psychological impact of biculturalism: evidence and theory. Psychol Bull 114(3):395–412, 1993
29. Jilek W: Traditional healing in the prevention and treatment of alcohol and drug abuse. Transcult Psychiatr Res Rev 31(3):219–258, 1994

5

Overview/Summary

It would be ideal for the purposes of presenting an overview of alcohol use and alcoholism in the United States to draw from studies that use a national sampling method to determine current and past drinking patterns in the majority white population, as well as in the four federally designated ethnic minority populations: African Americans, Hispanic Americans, Asian Americans and Pacific Islanders, and Native Americans. With such data, it would be possible to make detailed and precise comparisons among the four ethnic minority groups and between them and the majority population on fundamental issues of alcohol use and alcoholism. These comparisons would include lifetime prevalence of alcoholism in each group; comparative proportion of frequent heavy drinkers and of alcohol abstainers; peak age for alcohol abuse in each designated group; gender differences in alcohol use; and differences in drinking according to family income, family history of alcoholism, and mortality related directly and indirectly to alcohol abuse and dependence. Ideally, there should also be comparative data on the relationship between immigration status or generations of immigration and patterns of drinking. We have noted in the introduction of this book and in the chapters that focus on alcohol use in the designated ethnic minority populations, that we have not reached the ideal of comparably collected, nationally sampled data sets. On the other hand, sufficient data do exist to allow for direct comparisons on a number of those fundamental issues and for limited comparisons, or inferences, to be made. Making those comparisons is the purpose of this overview/summary chapter. In addition, we point out some of the policy implications of the findings in relation to the treatment and prevention of alcohol abuse and alcohol dependence in the four ethnic minority populations studied. We also briefly address areas of needed research that emerged from our review of the subject.

Lifetime Prevalence of Alcoholism

In the 1980s the national Epidemiologic Catchment Area (ECA) study collected sufficient data to make possible some of the direct comparisons referred to as the ideal situation. Data on the lifetime prevalence of alcoholism derived from ECA sources (1), shown in Table 5–1, for white, black, and Hispanic subjects reveal similar overall rates for whites and blacks and for both men and women. The lifetime alcoholism rates are comparatively higher for Hispanic men and slightly lower for Hispanic women. In each of these three populations, the lifetime risk of alcoholism is considerably higher for men than it is for women.

Considering next the prevalence of alcoholism by age, different patterns can be seen for the three groups. Alcoholism rates for whites, both men and women, peak in the 18- to 29-year age group. The rates fall progressively after age 30. Among black men, alcoholism rates are lowest in

Table 5–1. Lifetime prevalence of alcoholism

		Racial/ethnic group (%)		
Age (years)	**Gender**	**White**	**Black**	**Hispanic**
18–29	Male	28	13	30
	Female	8	4	5
30–44	Male	27	31	36
	Female	5	7	4
45–64	Male	20	33	26
	Female	3	7	3
65+	Male	13	22	18
	Female	1	2	1
Total	Male	23	24	30
	Female	5	5	4

Source. Adapted from Helzer JE, Burnam A, McEvory LT: "Alcohol Use and Dependence," in *Psychiatric Disorder in America.* Edited by Robins LN, Regier DA. New York, Free Press, 1991, pp 81–115.

those ages 18–29 but rise dramatically among black men ages 30–64, exceeding the alcoholism rates for white men of the same age. The lifetime alcoholism rates for black men over age 65 remain comparatively high. For Hispanic men, the peak of alcoholism is among those ages 30–44, but prevalence rates are very high in younger men as well, slightly exceeding those for white men ages 18–29 and more than twice the rates for black men in this age group. The data also show that Hispanic men have a higher lifetime prevalence of alcoholism than white men in all age categories and have higher rates than black men ages 18–44. However, alcoholism rates among black men over age 45 exceed those for both white and Hispanic men of similar age.

Lifetime prevalence rates of alcoholism in women are much lower than in men, but the pattern of age distribution is very similar—that is, among white women, alcoholism rates are highest in women ages 18–29, then fall progressively with increasing age (Table 5–1). The same pattern is seen among Hispanic women, but not among black women, in whom alcoholism rates are highest in those ages 30–64 (1).

In summary, the greatest risk of alcoholism among blacks, both men and women, is in the middle years (in the age groups 30–44 and 45–64, respectively). For Hispanic Americans, the risk is greatest in the age groups 18–29 and 30–44 for both men and women. For whites, the risk is greatest among those in the age group 18–29 for both men and women. The overall pattern for Hispanic men shows a higher risk of alcoholism than for white and black men, but a slightly lower risk for Hispanic women.

Frequent Heavy Drinking

Data from the National Household Survey of Health Status conducted in the mid-1980s enable comparisons among white, black, and Hispanic segments of the population concerning alcohol abuse—specifically, frequent heavy drinking (2). Table 5–2 shows that overall frequent heavy drinking prevalence rates are slightly higher in whites among both men and women.

There are differences in the pattern of frequent heavy drinking by age group, as there were with lifetime prevalence of alcoholism. Among white men, frequent heavy drinking occurs in the greatest numbers in the age group 18–29 and decreases progressively with age. By contrast, the peak rates of frequent heavy drinking are found in black men ages 50–59; this is also the case for lifetime alcoholism prevalence in black men. Black men ages 18–29 have much lower rates of frequent heavy drinking, as well as of lifetime prevalence of alcoholism, than white men

Table 5–2. Prevalence of frequent heavy drinking in different age groups

Age (years)	Gender	Racial/ethnic group (%)		
		White	Black	Hispanic
18–29	Male	31	16	17
	Female	7	6	2
30–39	Male	21	17	26
	Female	8	5	2
40–49	Male	19	14	11
	Female	7	6	2
50–59	Male	17	20	12
	Female	1	2	8
60+	Male	4	5	3
	Female	1	1	0
Total	Male	19	15	17
	Female	5	4	3

Source. Adapted from *U.S. Department of Health and Human Services: National Household Survey, 1984, Health Status and Minorities and Low Income Groups*, 3rd Edition. Washington, DC, U.S. Government Printing Office, 1991.

of the same age (3). Indeed, black men have lower rates of frequent heavy drinking than white men in all age groups below age 50 and somewhat higher rates than white men over age 50 (3).

There are also similarities in the patterns of frequent heavy drinking and of lifetime prevalence of alcoholism in Hispanic men, with peak risk occurring in men in their 30s (4). However, the risk of frequent heavy drinking in Hispanic men ages 18–29 is substantially less than their lifetime risk for alcoholism. It is only in the age category 30–39 that the rate of frequent heavy drinking among Hispanic men exceeds the rates for either white or black men of similar age (4, 5).

Comparable data sets for Asian Americans and Native Americans are not yet available, but limited data suggest that among some groups of Asian American men, in particular Japanese American and Korean American men in their 30s and 40s, rates of frequent heavy drinking may be quite similar to those of white and black men, whereas for younger and older men, rates are substantially lower (6). For Native American men ages 25–44, rates of frequent heavy drinking appear to be much higher than for white men of similar age, whereas rates for older Native American men are lower (7, 8).

As with lifetime prevalence of alcoholism, the overall prevalence rates for frequent heavy drinking among men are higher than those for women in each of the three ethnic groups for which data are available from the National Household Health Survey (2, 4). Among both white and black women, the rates of frequent heavy drinking do not vary greatly in women in their 20s, 30s, and 40s, but drop sharply among older women. White women in their 30s have substantially higher rates of frequent heavy drinking than black women. Hispanic women have much lower rates of frequent heavy drinking than white and black women, except for those age 50–59. Asian American women evidently also have very low rates of frequent heavy drinking, but this is not the case with Native American women, for whom binge drinking is a great problem among women in their 20s, as it is with Native American men in their 20s and 30s (9–11). Alcohol use drops sharply in older Native American women.

In summary, the patterns of frequent heavy drinking are similar to those for lifetime prevalence of alcoholism. Risk is highest among whites, both men and women, in the age group 18–29, for black men age 50–59, and for Hispanic men in their 30s. For Asian Americans, frequent heavy drinking occurs mostly in men in their 30s and 40s, and among Native Americans it is a major problem for men in their 20s and 30s. It is also a serious problem for Native American women of the same age.

Abstaining From Alcohol Use

Nondrinking is a subject that is often overlooked in discussions of alcohol use and alcoholism, especially among physicians whose focus, understandably, is on illness and disease. However, information about the prevalence of alcohol abstention in a given population provides counterbalance to an assessment of alcohol use that focuses almost exclusively on the deleterious legal, medical, and social consequences of excessive alcohol use.

Data derived from the National Household Health Survey, shown in Table 5–3, reveal higher alcohol abstinence rates among black subjects than whites (1). These differences are especially apparent for women. The pattern of abstinence among white subjects is generally the opposite of that for lifetime prevalence of alcoholism—that is, abstinence rates are lowest in the youngest group sampled (those ages 18–29) and increase progressively with increasing age. This pattern is quite clear for white women and for white men also, with the exception of those in their 30s.

Table 5–3. Prevalence of abstaining from alcohol in different age groups

Age (years)	Gender	Racial/ethnic group (%)		
		White	Black	Hispanic
18–29	Male	17	23	22
	Female	22	34	40
30–39	Male	13	15	17
	Female	30	32	45
40–49	Male	21	37	23
	Female	35	56	41
50–59	Male	30	29	24
	Female	35	60	47
60+	Male	41	60	30
	Female	49	69	78
Total	Male	24	29	22
	Female	34	46	47

Source. Adapted from Helzer JE, Burnam A, McEvory LT: "Alcohol Abuse and Dependence," in *Psychiatric Disorders in America.* Edited by Robins LN, Regier DA. New York, Free Press, 1991, pp. 81–115.

A different pattern is apparent for black subjects, in whom high abstinence rates in a given age group do not correspond with low lifetime prevalence rates for alcoholism in that age group, either for men or women. On the other hand, there is a striking difference between abstention rates for black women and those for white women: abstinence rates are much higher among black women in all age groups except those in their 30s (1, 12). The trend is similar, although much less striking, for black men, who show somewhat higher abstinence rates than white men in all age categories except those in their 50s (1).

Abstinence rates in Hispanic men are lowest for men in their 30s, among whom lifetime prevalence rates for alcoholism are highest. Abstinence rates for younger men, as well as for those in their 40s and 50s, are similar (1, 4). Abstinence rates for Hispanic women under age 40 and over age 60 are much higher than comparable rates for white and black women of similar ages. For women in their 40s and 50s, however, the highest rates of abstinence are found among black women (1, 12).

Among Asian Americans, overall abstinence rates appear to be approximately twice as high as those for whites. This overall finding applies for both men and women, with the differences being more striking for women (6, 9). Abstinence rates have been found to be high among older Asian American women. For Native Americans, overall abstinence rates are believed to be substantially lower than for whites for both men and women younger than 40 (10, 11). On the other hand, abstinence rates among Native Americans in the older age categories are probably higher than those in whites of similar age (7, 8).

To summarize the findings on abstinence, the most generalizable point is the greater prevalence of abstinence in the ethnic minority populations, especially among women. Abstinence rates tend to increase with age, and this pattern is seen most clearly with white women. Low rates of abstinence in a given age group tend to correlate with high rates of lifetime alcoholism, and high rates of abstinence correlate with low lifetime rates of alcoholism.

Family History of Alcoholism

A study of positive and negative family history of alcoholism in a representative sample of whites, African Americans, Hispanic Americans, Asian Americans, and Native Americans has provided extremely useful comparative data on this subject (13). The data, shown in Table 5–4, indicate that Native Americans have the highest rates of positive family history of alcoholism among both male and female subjects. Rates for whites, both male and female, are marginally higher than those for African Americans. Rates for Hispanic Americans are somewhat lower than those for African Americans. Asian American subjects have dramatically lower rates of positive family history of alcoholism than do other racial/ethnic groups. The rates for Native Americans are much higher than for all other groups.

Table 5–4. Positive family history of alcoholism

Racial/ethnic group	Men (%)	Women (%)
White	37[a]	40[a]
African American	34	36
Hispanic American	27	32
Asian American	12	16
Native American	46	63

[a]Age-adjusted, weighted percentage figures.
Source. Adapted from Harford TC: "Family History of Alcholism in the United States: Prevalence and Demographic Characteristics." *British Journal of Addiction* 87:931–935, 1992.

Alcohol-Related Mortality

It has been estimated that patients with alcoholism have an overall mortality rate from all causes directly and indirectly related to alcohol abuse and alcohol dependence that is more than twice as high as that for nonalcoholic persons. In the category of alcohol-induced causes of death, rates for African Americans are nearly three times as high as the rates for whites among both men and women (14, 15). For Native Americans, these rates rise even higher, to approximately four times the rates for whites. Again, this is the case for both men and women. On the other hand, alcohol-related mortality rates for Asian Americans are much lower than for the other population groups.

Table 5–5 presents data on alcohol-related mortality for men. In addition to mortality directly related to alcohol dependence and alcohol abuse, summarized previously, a similar pattern is evident for alcoholic liver disease, principally cirrhosis—that is, the death rate for Native American men is nearly three times and for African American men nearly twice as high as it is for white men, whereas for Asian American men the rate is only one-third of the death rate for white men (15). For non-alcohol–related liver disease, on the other hand, differences in mortality rates between ethnic groups are much less divergent.

Causes of death that are indirectly related to alcohol abuse and alcohol dependence include motor vehicle accidents, falls, boating accidents, homicide, and suicide. It is estimated that about half of all motor

Table 5–5. Male alcohol-related mortality rates: 1980[a]

	Racial/ethnic group			
Cause of death	**White**	**African American**	**Asian American[b]**	**Native American**
Alcohol dependence	11	29	2	39
Alcohol abuse	3	6	1	16
Alcoholic liver disease	9	15	3	25
Other liver disease	21	28	10	28
Motor vehicle accidents	36	31	15	75
Homicide	11	66	18	23
Suicide	20	10	11	21

[a]Per 100,000 population.
[b]Estimated figures.
Source. Adapted from U.S. Mortality Statistics, 1980, p. 445.

vehicle accidents, falls, boating accidents, and homicides are alcohol related, and a substantial percentage of suicides also involve excessive alcohol intake. The data in Table 5–5 show that although suicide rates among African American men are much lower than those for white men and fatal motor vehicle accident rates for African American men are substantially lower, homicide rates are six times higher than for white men.

The mortality rates for Asian American men show a different pattern; low suicide and motor vehicle death rates compared with white men, but higher homicide rates. Among Native American men, the rate of motor vehicle deaths is more than double that for other racial/ethnic groups, the homicide rate is twice as high as for white men but much lower than for blacks, and the suicide rate is similar to that for whites.

Migration, Immigration, Acculturation, Alcohol Use, and Alcoholism

Some intriguing findings have been presented in the preceding chapters relating to alcohol use among migrants and immigrants to the United States, compared with people who are the children or grandchildren of immigrants. Other studies have compared alcohol use in rural areas and urban settings.

With respect to immigration and by inference, the effects of acculturative stress on alcohol use and abuse, one study found that among Mexican American men, the percentage of subjects who reported daily alcohol consumption was much higher for third-generation immigrants than it was for first- and second-generation immigrants (16). The comparable rate for a control sample of Mexican men living in Mexico was much lower than for Mexican American immigrant men. Although the pattern of *daily* alcohol use increased in each generation of Mexican American men, *monthly* alcohol use decreased. The same pattern of increased daily and decreased monthly drinking is also seen in Mexican American women.

In another study of frequent heavy drinking and abstention among Mexican migrants, frequent heavy drinking rates were highest and alcohol abstention rates lowest among Mexican men who had migrated to the United States within the preceding 5 years (17).

Another study that addressed differences in alcohol use as related to immigrant status compared overall frequency of drinking between Japanese living in Japan and Japanese Americans living in Hawaii (mainly first-generation immigrants) and in California (mainly third-generation immigrants) (9). Both male and female samples were included. The findings were similar for both men and women; Japanese Americans drank less and abstained more than Japanese living in Japan and whites in the United States. There were no significant differences according to generation of immigrant status in the United States.

Several studies among the Native American population support the proposition that urban migration carries a high risk of increasing alcohol abuse, along with discrimination and unemployment and erosion of self-esteem—all factors that have been clearly shown to be associated with increased alcohol use (18, 19).

The issue of urban versus rural differences in alcohol abuse and alcohol dependence was examined in one component of the ECA study (20). In that study it was found that black men living in rural areas had higher rates of alcoholism than black men living in urban areas. These differences were not clearly evident for black women or for white men or women.

In summary, no clear association emerges from the studies of migration to the United States or of immigrant status across generations in relation to alcohol use, except for the case of Hispanic Americans. There is considerable variation across racial/ethnic groups. Urban migration does seem to be associated with increased alcohol use and abuse, but here, too, there is considerable variance within and between racial/ethnic groups.

Intragroup Variation

In each of the chapters concerned with alcohol use and alcoholism in the four ethnic minority populations, we have emphasized the diversity within each designated population. There is great intragroup variation in history of immigration to the United States; internal migration and settlement patterns within the country; and differences in socioeconomic status, religion, language use, educational experiences, social integration, and responses to acculturative stress. All of these factors have a bearing on intragroup differences in alcohol use and alcoholism.

We review some of those intragroup variations here to give them further emphasis. In the chapter devoted to Hispanic Americans, data on lifetime prevalence of alcoholism were presented first for the total Hispanic population in comparison with the white population of the United States. The same type of comparisons were made for frequent heavy drinking and for abstaining in the two population groups. Thereafter, data on lifetime prevalence of alcoholism were presented only for Mexican Americans and whites in the Los Angeles component of the national ECA study. Next, comparisons were made between three of the largest subpopulations of Hispanic people in the United States: Mexican Americans, Puerto Rican Americans living in the mainland United States, and Cuban Americans. This analysis revealed some significant differences between these groups. With respect to frequent heavy drinking, it was shown that rates for Mexican American and Puerto Rican American men were similar and much higher than comparative rates for Cuban American men. Frequent heavy drinking was found to be very uncommon in all three groups of Hispanic women, and alcohol abstinence rates were very high. Among Hispanic men, abstinence rates were highest in the Puerto Rican group and substantially lower among Mexican Americans.

Similar intragroup comparative data were presented in the chapter on Asian Americans. These data showed that frequent heavy drinking occurred to a much greater extent among Japanese American and Korean American men than among Chinese American men; that Japanese American women were the only group of Asian American women to have substantial numbers of frequent heavy drinkers; that infrequent drinking and alcohol abstinence rates were highest among Korean Americans, both men and women; and that infrequent drinking/abstinence occurred at much higher rates among Korean American and Chinese American women than among Japanese American women.

The chapter on African Americans reviewed some data from the ECA study that compared alcoholism rates between those living in urban areas and rural areas. Alcoholism rates were higher among African American men in rural areas; this was true for all age group comparisons. These differences were not found among African American women.

Among Native Americans, studies have demonstrated marked intragroup or tribal variation in attitudes toward alcohol use, rates of alcoholism, frequent heavy drinking, and alcohol abstention. Chapter 4 included references to such variation; for example, Navajo acceptance of social drinking, especially among younger men, as normative, in contrast to the Hopi, who view drinking as irresponsible and a threat to their religious principles (21). Concerning heavy drinking, prevalence rates have been found to vary greatly between tribes, from 14% among the Navajo in the Southwest to 26% for the Ute tribe in Colorado and 42% among the Ojibwa in Wisconsin and Minnesota. A number of studies have demonstrated that heavy drinking rates are substantially higher among Native Americans living in urban areas than in those in rural areas, mainly on tribal reservations. For example, among Native Americans living in the Los Angeles area, the rate of heavy drinking was found to be 16%, compared with a rate of 6% for Native Americans living in rural areas in California (18). In this chapter, we also described the use of alcohol for ritual purposes and as part of religious observances in certain Native American tribes, whereas use of alcohol for other purposes and in other contexts is strongly discouraged. The proportion of Native American tribal members who belong to religious organizations that prohibit alcohol use (e.g., Seventh Day Adventists) has grown steadily since the 1970s.

Income and Drinking Patterns

The relationship between family income and alcohol use is particularly complex, not only between racial/ethnic groups, but also within ethnic groups. The studies of these relationships have produced seemingly contradictory findings.

As noted in Chapter 1, the highest rates of frequent heavy drinking were found among African American men in the middle income group. By contrast, frequent heavy drinking rates among white men were at their peak among men in the highest income group and also very high among those in the lowest income category (3). The association between low income and high alcohol use was found not to apply to black men in the way that it did for white men.

The strongest association between income and alcohol use has been found in Hispanic Americans, especially among women. The rates of alcohol abstention among Hispanic American women have been noted to decrease progressively with increasing levels of income, while rates of frequent heavy drinking increased (4). Some similarities in this pattern were noted for Hispanic American men, although a clear association was apparent only for men with an annual income of more than $30,000, whose rates of abstention were much lower and whose rates of frequent heavy drinking were much higher than men with lower income levels.

Studies of the relationship between income and alcohol use are not yet available for Asian Americans and Native Americans. However, some inferences can be drawn from available information. The association between increasing income and increasing alcohol use is clearest among Japanese Americans, the majority of whom have been living in the United States for two or more generations and whose income levels exceed those of other Asian American ethnic groups. In the case of Japanese Americans, it has been observed that overall rates of alcohol abstention are lower and frequent heavy drinking rates are higher than corresponding rates for other Asian American groups.

With respect to Native Americans, available data point to a strong association between frequent heavy drinking and low income/high unemployment, especially in urban areas.

Summary Points

1. Overall lifetime prevalence rates for alcoholism are similar for white and African American men and women, higher for Hispanic American men, and slightly lower for Hispanic American women.
2. Lifetime risk of alcoholism is considerably higher for men than for women. This is equally true for white, African American, and Hispanic American population groups.
3. Highest rates of alcoholism occur in white men ages 18–29, in African American men ages 45–64, and in Hispanic American men ages 30–44. For Asian American men, alcoholism rates peak in mid-adulthood (ages 30–60), and in Native American men the peak occurs in youth and young adulthood (ages 16–18 to 25–29).
4. The overall pattern of lifetime prevalence of alcoholism in women is similar to the pattern for men in each racial/ethnic group. Rates are highest in white women ages 18–29, African American women ages 30–64, and Native American women in youth and young adulthood (ages 16–18 to 25–29). Hispanic American women are an exception, with alcoholism rates peaking in those ages 18–29.
5. Overall rates of frequent heavy drinking are similar among whites, African Americans, and Hispanic Americans, but the peak risk differs by age group. Highest rates of frequent heavy drinking occur in white men in youth and young adulthood, African American men in their 50s, Hispanic American men in their 30s, and Asian American men in their 30s and 40s. Rates for Native American men remain comparatively high from youth through mid-adulthood (ages 16–18 to 25–29).
6. Frequent heavy drinking occurs about four times more often among men than women. In women, overall rates are probably highest among Native Americans, followed by white, African American, Hispanic American, and Asian American women, in descending frequency.
7. Overall prevalence rates of alcohol abstention are higher in the ethnic minority populations than among the white majority, and this distinction is especially clear among women.
8. Very large scale differences in prevalence rates between men and women are not encountered for alcohol abstention, in contrast to

the findings for lifetime prevalence of alcoholism and for frequent heavy drinking, except in the case of Asian Americans.

9. Striking differences in alcohol abstention are found between white and African American women, in that abstinence rates are much higher among African American women in nearly every age category.
10. Family history of alcoholism is highest among Native Americans, both men and women, followed by whites, African Americans, Hispanic Americans, and Asian Americans.
11. Mortality rates directly and indirectly related to alcohol consumption are much higher in United States ethnic minority groups than in the white majority population, with the exception of Asian Americans.
12. Death rates for alcohol dependence, alcohol abuse, and alcoholic liver disease among African Americans and Native Americans range from twice to five times as high as comparable rates for whites.
13. There is a great deal of intragroup variation with respect to alcohol use, alcohol abuse, and alcohol dependence in each of the four major racial/ethnic groups, as well as within the white majority population.
14. There is a great need for studies of alcohol use and alcohol-related problems in the ethnic minority populations of the United States that utilize comparable definitions of terms, nationally distributed study samples, and similar research designs and strategies for data analysis and that take into account intragroup variation.

Policy Implications for Treatment and Prevention

In the preceding sections of this chapter, we have provided an overview of major findings on lifetime prevalence of alcoholism in the United States, as well as peak prevalence rates for lifetime alcoholism and frequent heavy drinking according to age and gender. We have reviewed the findings on these topics for the white majority population and made comparisons, to the extent the data allow, with African Americans, Hispanic Americans, Asian Americans, and Native Americans. We have given an overview of available information on alcohol abstinence, family history of alcoholism, urban and rural differences in alcohol use, and the relationship between urban migration and immigration status and alcohol use, as well as income level and alcohol use. We have included summary analyses of each of these topics. We turn now to some descriptive features of the population receiving treatment for alcohol- and drug-related illnesses.

Given that lifetime prevalence of alcoholism as well as frequent heavy drinking occur in men to a much greater extent than in women, it is not surprising that 72% of all people treated for alcohol-related disorders are men, even though men make up only about 50% of the total national population. It is also not surprising that more than 50% of people treated for alcohol-related disorders consist of those ages 25–44, in view of the high prevalence rates of lifetime alcoholism in that age group (22).

However, the distribution of the treatment population according to racial/ethnic composition is surprising. White patients are underrepresented in the population of those being treated for alcohol-related illnesses compared with their proportionate numbers in the national population, whereas the minority population is overrepresented. This is particularly true for African American and Hispanic American patients, whose numbers in the treatment population are approximately twice as high as their representation in the national population (22). Given the comparatively low prevalence of alcohol-related illness in the Asian American population and the comparatively high prevalence of such illness among Native Americans, we could infer that this constitutes an overrepresentation of Native Americans in the treatment population for alcohol-related illness.

Thus, it would appear that a large amount of treatment is directed toward alcohol-related illness in the minority populations, especially African American and Hispanic American patients. In considering the significance of these findings, it is important to recall that overall lifetime prevalence rates for alcoholism are similar for white and African American populations and that prevalence rates for frequent heavy drinking are lower among African Americans than among whites. For Hispanic Americans, overall rates of lifetime prevalence of alcoholism are higher in men than comparable figures for white and African American men.

Consider next the data on mortality directly related to alcohol—that is, deaths caused by alcohol dependence, alcohol abuse, and alcoholic liver cirrhosis, which are approximately two to five times higher in the ethnic minority populations, especially African Americans and Native Americans, than in whites. The picture that is revealed by these data is that despite their overrepresentation in the treatment population, the ethnic minority population experiences a much higher death rate from alcohol-related illnesses.

Several other points should be emphasized that have policy implications for treatment and prevention strategies for alcohol-related illnesses in the ethnic minority populations. One of the most robust findings of our review of alcohol use and abuse in the ethnic minority populations is that alcohol abuse is a much greater problem among men than women, when compared with the majority white population. Also, the peak age of risk for alcoholism in the ethnic minority populations differs significantly from that in the white population, which has peak risk in youth and young adulthood, compared with young and mid-adulthood in the ethnic minority populations. There are, in addition, some important findings in the area of alcohol use related to income, suggesting that there is a trend toward increased alcohol consumption and decreased abstinence with increasing income levels in the ethnic minority populations.

Drawing together all of these findings, the following policy approaches to treatment and prevention offer promise of reducing alcohol-related morbidity and mortality in the ethnic minority populations:

1. Greater emphasis on early detection of alcohol abuse and alcohol dependence to institute early diagnosis and treatment aimed at secondary prevention—that is, an approach that would involve reversibility of illness and avoid end-stage disease.
2. Greater emphasis on intervention with the high-risk segments of ethnic minority populations—those subgroups with the highest rates of frequent heavy drinking: especially African Americans, both men and women, in mid-adulthood; Hispanic American men in their 30s; Asian Americans, especially Japanese Americans, in mid-adulthood; and Native Americans, both men and women, in youth and young adulthood. In this and the preceding area, screening for alcoholism in primary care settings should be done as a routine procedure.
3. Greater emphasis on recognition of the comparatively high rates of alcohol abstention in the ethnic minority population, especially among women, to target alcohol abstention and moderate alcohol use as culturally acceptable, normative approaches to alcohol use.
4. Active public health prevention programs aimed at increasing awareness of the risks and consequences of heavy drinking and alcoholism. Such approaches have proven to be highly effective in changing attitudes and behaviors concerning smoking since the 1970s. Once again, the priority targets of these efforts should be those groups at the greatest risk for alcohol abuse and with the highest alcoholism prevalence rates described in this report. These prevention programs should range from grassroots efforts and community coalitions to national campaigns.

5. Reduction of social disorganization and enhancement of individual and communal self-esteem through increased education and decreased unemployment, underemployment, and cultural stereotyping.

Policy Implications for Research

Two interdigitating approaches are needed as a first step to fill important gaps in available information and knowledge about alcohol use and alcohol abuse in the ethnic minority populations. Most critical is the need to identify systematically the ethnic minority populations in the national population, specifically by identifying them as separate groups in the collection of national census data and in national surveys of health and illness. The national ECA study represents a model of research design in this regard because of its intentional oversampling of African Americans and Hispanic Americans in several of the study sites—even though similar oversampling was not done for Asian Americans and Native Americans. The ECA study design is also to be commended for its inclusion of urban and rural differences, although it failed to include generational differences in immigrant status as a variable of interest. The inclusion of all of these variables would greatly enhance our ability to take account of similarities and differences in incidence, prevalence, treatment, and prevention of illnesses within the diverse groups that make up the United States population.

At the same time there continues to be a great need for highly focused, emic or community-based studies of defined populations (e.g., Southeast Asians living in southern New England, Puerto Ricans living in New York City, Mexican Americans living in Los Angeles, Native Americans living in Denver or Los Angeles, or African Americans living in rural Georgia or in urban New Orleans). Such studies would be focused enough to determine community norms in attitudes and behaviors related to ethnic identification, health-seeking practices, and responses to treatment, as well as specifics of alcohol use, abstention, frequent heavy drinking, and alcoholism. These kinds of emic studies could be sufficiently finely focused to take account of the kind of intragroup variations that are important in avoiding stereotyping of any population.

The summary points outlined in this chapter suggest several specific areas for further research that should be pursued as a matter of policy because of their potential for reducing alcoholism. These include studies of factors determining gender, age, and ethnic differences in lifetime prevalence and risk of alcoholism and frequent heavy drinking, as well as differences in alcohol abstention rates. The causative factors may be biological, psychological, or sociocultural in nature and may act interdependently, reflecting cultural differences in normative behavior and coping styles. Identifying these factors could, in turn, lead to culturally sensitive treatment and prevention projects for specific population groups.

Another area of potentially important research involves the factors leading to comparatively high alcohol-related mortality rates, particularly among African Americans and Hispanic Americans, despite their having lifetime prevalence rates of alcoholism similar to those of whites. Native Americans also have disproportionately high alcohol-related mortality rates. These bio-psycho-sociocultural factors may include genetic predisposition, nutrition and dietary patterns, access to health care, socioeconomic status, and educational background, among other factors.

Intragroup variation is another needed area of research. This has to do with the heterogeneity of the racial/ethnic groups, which adds yet another level of complexity to efforts to understand alcohol use and alcoholism among them. Therefore, research projects that focus on adequately representative samples of specific population groups, analyzing issues as dissimilar as genetic pedigree, interpersonal behavioral patterns, and extent of acculturative stress are needed.

Alcohol use is a phenomenon deeply imbued with value judgments and stereotypes. Alcohol use in racial/ethnic minority populations is, we contend, a subject that is even more imbued with value judgments and cultural stereotyping and is, accordingly, a particularly apt subject for study using both etic and emic approaches and employing interdisciplinary teams of investigators.

References

1. Helzer JE, Burnam A, McEvory LT: Alcohol abuse and dependence, in Psychiatric Disorders in America. Edited by Robins LN, Regier DA. New York, Free Press, 1991, pp 81–115
2. U.S. Department of Health and Human Services: National Household Survey, 1984, Health Status of Minorities and Low Income Groups, 3rd Edition. Washington, DC, U.S. Government Printing Office, 1991
3. Herd D: Subgroup differences in drinking patterns among black and white men: results from a national survey. J Stud Alcohol 51: 221–232, 1990
4. Caetano R: Drinking patterns and alcohol problems in a national sample of U.S. Hispanics, in Alcohol Use Among U.S. Ethnic Minorities (Research Monograph No 18). Edited by Spiegler D, Tate D,

Aitken S, et al (DHHS Publ No ADM-89-1435). Washington, DC, U.S. Government Printing Office, 1989, pp 147–162

5. Alcohol Drug Abuse and Mental Health Administration: National Clearinghouse for Alcohol and Drug Information. Update, January 1989
6. Chi I, Lubben JE, Kitano HH: Differences in drinking behavior among three Asian American groups. J Stud Alcohol 50(1):15–23, 1989
7. Leland JH: Native American alcohol use: a review of the literature, in Tulapai to Tokay. Edited by Mail P, McDonald D. New Haven, CT, HRAF Press, 1980, pp 1–56
8. Lemert EM: Drinking among American Indians, in Alcohol, Science and Society Revisited. Edited by Gomberg E, White H, Carpenter J. Ann Arbor, University of Michigan Press, 1982, pp 80–95
9. Kono H, Towle LH, Harford TC: Alcohol Consumption Patterns and Related Problems in the United States and Japan. Rockville, MD, National Institute of Alcohol Abuse and Alcoholism, 1991
10. Blum R, Harmon B, Harris L, et al: American Indian-Alaska Native youth health. JAMA 267:1637–1644, 1992
11. Oetting E, Beauvais F: Epidemiology and correlates of alcohol use among Indian adolescents living on reservations, in Alcohol Use Among United States Ethnic Minorities (Research Monograph No 18). Edited by Spiegler D, Tate D, Aitken S, et al (DHHS Publ No ADM-89-1435). Washington, DC, U.S. Government Printing Office, 1989, pp 239–267
12. Lillie-Blanton M, MacKenzie E, Anthony JC: Black-white differences in alcohol use by women: Baltimore survey findings. Public Health Rep 106:124–133, 1991
13. Harford TC: Family history of alcoholism in the United States: prevalence and demographic characteristics. Br J Addict 87:931–935, 1992
14. Monthly Vital Statistics Report 41(suppl 7):28–38, 1993
15. United States Mortality Statistics, 1980, p 445
16. Gilbert MJ: Alcohol-related practices, problems, and norms among Mexican Americans: an overview, in Alcohol Use Among U.S. Ethnic Minorities (Research Monograph No 18). Edited by Spiegler D, Tate D, Aitken S, et al (DHHS Publ No ADM-89-1435). Washington, DC, U.S. Government Printing Office, 1989, pp 115–134
17. Caetano R, Medina Mora ME: Acculturation and drinking among people of Mexican descent in Mexico and the United States. J Stud Alcohol 49:462–471, 1988

18. Weibel-Orlando J, Weisner T, Long J: Urban and rural Indian drinking patterns: implications for intervention and policy development. Subst Alcohol Action Misuse 5:45–57, 1984
19. Beltrame T, McQueen D: Urban and rural Indian drinking patterns: the special case of the Lumbee. Int J Addict 14:533–548, 1979
20. Blazer D, Crowell BA Jr, George LK: Alcohol abuse and dependence in the rural south. Arch Gen Psychiatry 44:736–740, 1987
21. Levy JE, Kunitz S: Indian Drinking: Navaho Practices and Anglo-American Theories. New York, Wiley, 1974
22. Holzer J, Canino G (eds): Alcoholism in North America, Europe and Asia. London, England, Oxford University Press, 1992

GAP Committees and Membership

Committee on Adolescence

Lois Flaherty, Bluebell, PA, *Chairperson*
Ian A. Canino, New York, NY
Warren J. Gadpaille, Denver, CO
Harvey Horowitz, Philadelphia, PA
Sarah Huertas-Goldman, San Juan, PR
Paulina F. Kernberg, New York, NY
Clarice J. Kestenbaum, New York, NY
Silvio J. Onesti, Jr., Belmont, MA

Committee on Aging

Gene D. Cohen, Washington, DC, *Chairperson*
Karen Blank, West Hartford, CT
Charles M. Gaitz, Houston, TX
Ira R. Katz, Philadelphia, PA
Andrew F. Leuchter, Los Angeles, CA
Gabe J. Maletta, Minneapolis, MN
Richard A. Margolin, Nashville, TN
Kenneth M. Sakauye, New Orleans, LA
Charles A. Shamoian, Larchmont, NY

Committee on Alcoholism and the Addictions

John A. Menninger, Denver, CO, *Chairperson*
Stephen Dilts, Denver, CO
Richard J. Frances, Newark, NJ
William Frosch, New York, NY
Marc Galanter, New York, NY
Collins E. Lewis, St. Louis, MO
Earl A. Loomis, Jr., Augusta, GA
Robert Millman, New York, NY
Edgar P. Nace, Dallas, TX
Sally Satel, Lafayette Hill, PA
Richard Suchinsky, Silver Spring, MD
John S. Tamerin, Greenwich, CT
Joseph Westermeyer, Minneapolis, MN
Doug Ziedonis, New Haven, CT

Committee on Child Psychiatry

Peter Jensen, *Co-Chairperson*
David A. Mrazek, Denver, CO, *Co-Chairperson*
William R. Beardslee, Woburn, MA
James M. Bell, Canaan, NY
Harlow Donald Dunton, New York, NY
John F. McDermott, Jr., Honolulu, HI
Cynthia R. Pfeffer, White Plains, NY
John Schowalter, New Haven, CT
Theodore Shapiro, New York, NY
Peter E. Tanguay, Los Angeles, CA
Leonore Terr, San Francisco, CA

Committee on College StudentS

Earle Silber, Chevy Chase, MD, *Chairperson*
Robert L. Arnstein, Hamden, CT
Varda Backus, La Jolla, CA
Harrison P. Eddy, New York, NY
Myron B. Liptzin, Chapel Hill, NC
Malkah Tolpin Notman, Brookline, MA
Elizabeth Aub Reid, Cambridge, MA
Lorraine D. Siggins, New Haven, CT

Tom G. Stauffer, White Plains, NY
Robert Wenger, Philadelphia, PA

Committee on Cultural Psychiatry

Ezra Griffith, New Haven, CT, *Chairperson*
Renato Alarcon, Decatur, GA
Irma Bland, New Orleans, LA
Edward Foulks, New Orleans, LA
Francis Lu, San Francisco, CA
Maria Oquendo, San Antonio, TX
Pedro Ruiz, Houston, TX
Jose Arturo Silva, San Antonio, TX
Joe Yamamoto, Los Angeles, CA

Committee on Disabilities

Meyer S. Gunther, Chicago, IL, *Chairperson*
Bryan King, Los Angeles, CA
Robert S. Nesheim, Duluth, MN
William H. Sack, Portland, OR
William A. Sonis, Philadelphia, PA
Margaret L. Stuber, Los Angeles, CA
Henry H. Work, Bethesda, MD

Committee on the Family

Frederick Gottlieb, Los Angeles, CA, *Chairperson*
W. Robert Beavers, Dallas, TX
Lee Combrinck-Graham, Stamford, CT
James Griffith, Vienna, VA
Henry U. Grunebaum, Cambridge, MA
Herta A. Guttman, Montreal, PQ
Ann L. Price, Avon, CT
Lois Slovik, Boston, MA

Committee on Government Policy

Thomas L. Clannon, San Francisco, CA, *Chairperson*
Seymour Applebaum, Kew Garden, NY
Naomi Heller, Washington, DC

Roger Peele, Washington, DC
John P. D. Shemo, Charlottesville, VA
William W. Van Stone, Washington, DC

Committee on Human Sexuality

Bertram H. Schaffner, New York, NY, *Chairperson*
Paul L. Adams, Louisville, KY
Debra Carter, Portland, OR
Jack Drescher, New York, NY
Richard Friedman, New York, NY
Joan A. Lang, Galveston, TX
Harris B. Peck, New Rochelle, NY

Committee on International Relations

Vamik D. Volkan, Charlottesville, VA, *Chairperson*
Salman Akhtar, Philadelphia, PA
Letha B. Cole, Houston, TX
Robert M. Dorn, El Macero, CA
David R. Hawkins, Chapel Hill, NC
John S. Kafka, Washington, DC
Otto F. Kernberg, White Plains, NY
Peter A. Olsson, Houston, TX
Rita R. Rogers, Palos Verdes Estates, CA
Stephen B. Shanfield, San Antonio, TX
Edward Shapiro, Stockbridge, MA

Committee on Medical Education

Steven L. Dubovsky, Denver, CO, *Chairperson*
Leah Dickstein, Louisville, KY
Glen O. Gabbard, Topeka, KS
Saul I. Harrison, Torrance, CA
Harold I. Lief, Philadelphia, PA
Carol C. Nadelson, Boston, MA
Carolyn B. Robinowitz, Washington, DC
Stephen C. Scheiber, Deerfield, IL
James Scully, Washington, DC
Sidney L. Werkman, Washington, DC

Committee on Mental Health Services

W. Walter Menninger, Topeka, KS, *Chairperson*
Mary Jane England, Roseland, NJ
Richard Lippincott, McMinnville, OR
James Sabin, Boston, MA
Jose Maria Santiago, Tucson, AZ
Steven S. Sharfstein, Baltimore, MD
Altha Stewart, Philadelphia, PA
Michael Vergare, Philadelphia, PA
Jack A. Wolford, Pittsburgh, PA

Committee on Occupational Psychiatry

David B. Robbins, Chappaqua, NY, *Chairperson*
Peter L. Brill, Radnor, PA
Barrie S. Greiff, Newton, MA
Duane Q. Hagen, St. Louis, MO
Robert Larsen, San Francisco, CA
David E. Morrison, Palatine, IL
Jay B. Rohrlich, New York, NY
Clarence J. Rowe, St. Paul, MN

Committee on Planning and Communications

Robert W. Gibson, Towson, MD, *Chairperson*
Allan Beigel, Tucson, AZ
Doyle I. Carson, Dallas, TX
Robert S. Garber, Longboat Key, FL
Harvey L. Ruben, New Haven, CT
Melvin Sabshin, Washington, DC
Michael R. Zales, Tucson, AZ

Committee on Preventive Psychiatry

Naomi Rae-Grant, London, ON, *Chairperson*
Brian J. McConville, Cincinnati, OH
David R. Offord, Hamilton, ON
Morton M. Silverman, Chicago, IL
Hans Steiner, Palo Alto, CA
Warren T. Vaughan, Jr., Portola Valley, CA

Committee on Psychiatry and the Community

David G. Greenfield, Guilford, CT, *Chairperson*
C. Knight Aldrich, Charlottesville, VA
Francine Cournos, New York, NY
Stephen Goldfinger, Boston, MA
H. Richard Lamb, Los Angeles, CA
Kenneth Minkoff, Woburn, MA
John C. Nemiah, Hanover, NH
David Pollack, Portland, OR
John J. Schwab, Louisville, KY
John A. Talbott, Baltimore, MD
Allan Tasman, Louisville, KY

Committee on Psychiatry and the Law

Joseph Satten, San Francisco, CA, *Chairperson*
J. Richard Ciccone, Rochester, NY
Jeffrey Janofsky, Timonium, MD
Carl P. Malmquist, Minneapolis, MN
Jeffrey Metzner, Denver, CO
Betty Pfefferbaum, Oklahoma City, OK
Jonas R. Rappeport, Baltimore, MD
Phillip J. Resnick, Cleveland, OH
William D. Weitzel, Lexington, KY

Committee on Psychiatry and Religion

Richard C. Lewis, New Haven, CT, *Chairperson*
Naleen N. Andrade, Honolulu, HI
Keith G. Meador, Nashville, TN
Abigail R. Ostow, Belmont, MA
Sally K. Severino, White Plains, NY
Clyde R. Snyder, Fayetteville, NC
Herzl Spiro, Milwaukee, WI
Edwin R. Wallace IV, Augusta, GA

Committee on Psychopathology

Kathleen Pajer, Pittsburgh, PA, *Chairperson*
David A. Adler, Boston, MA

Jeffrey Berlant, Boise, ID
Lisa Dixon, Baltimore, MD
John P. Docherty, Nashua, NH
Robert A. Dorwart, Cambridge, MA
James M. Ellison, Watertown, MA
Samuel G. Siris, Glen Oaks, NY

Committee on Public Education

Steven E. Katz, New York, NY, *Chairperson*
David Baron, Ambler, PA
Jack W. Bonner III, Greenville, SC
Jeffrey L. Geller, Worcester, MA
Jeanne Leventhal, Hayward, CA
David Preven, New York, NY
Elise K. Richman, Scarsdale, NY
Boris G. Rifkin, Branford, CT
Andrew E. Slaby, Summit, NJ
Calvin R. Sumner, Buckhannon, WV
Laurence Tancredi New York, NY

Committee on Research

Zebulon Taintor, New York, NY, *Chairperson*
Robert Cancro, New York, NY
Russell Gardner, Galveston, TX
John H. Greist, Madison, WI
Jerry M. Lewis, Dallas, TX
John G. Looney, Durham, NC

Committee on Social Issues

Martha J. Kirkpatrick, Los Angeles, CA, *Chairperson*
Ian E. Alger, New York, NY
Roderic Gorney, Los Angeles, CA
H. James Lurie, Seattle, WA
Ted Nadelson, Boston, MA
Perry Ottenberg, Philadelphia, PA
Jane Rosenthal, New York, NY
Miriam Rosenthal, Cleveland, OH

Committee on Therapeutic Care

Alan Gruenberg, Philadelphia, PA, *Chairperson*
Thomas E. Curtis, Chapel Hill, NC
Donald C. Fidler, Morgantown, WV
Donald W. Hammersley, Washington, DC
William B. Hunter III, Albuquerque, NM
Milton Kramer, Cincinnati, OH
John Lipkin, Perry Point, MA
Robert E. Switzer, Dunn Loring, VA

Committee on Therapy

Susan Lazar, Washington, DC, *Chairperson*
Gerald Adler, Boston, MA
Jules R. Bemporad, White Plains, NY
Eugene B. Feigelson, Brooklyn, NY
Andrew P. Morrison, Cambridge, MA
William C. Offenkrantz, Scottsdale, AZ
Allan D. Rosenblatt, La Jolla, CA
Robert Waldinger, West Newton, MA

GINSBURG FELLOWS

Arlener Artis-Trower, Silver Spring, MD *(Committee on Therapeutic Care)*
Elizabeth C. Druss, Cambridge, MA *(Committee on Psychopathology)*
Louis Michel Elie, LaSalle, Quebec, Canada *(Committee on Aging)*
Ryan Finkenbine, Charleston, SC *(Committee on Social Issues)*
Risa Fishman, New York, NY *(Committee on Alcoholism and the Addictions)*
Anna Lucy Fitzgerald, Brighton, MA *(Committee on Cultural Psychiatry)*
Michael Golding, Carrboro, NC *(Committee on Government Policy)*
Scott A. Haas, Louisville, KY *(Committee on Psychiatry and the Law)*
Jacqueline Haimes, Silver Spring, MD *(Committee on Planning and Communications)*
Samia Hasan, Baltimore, MD *(Committee on College Students)*
Lyudmila Karlin, Great Neck, NY *(Committee on Psychiatry and the Community)*
Vassilis Koliatsos, Baltimore, MD *(Committee on Research)*

Heather Krell, Philadelphia, PA *(Committee on Disabilities)*
Patricia Lester, San Francisco, CA *(Committee on Adolescence)*
Mercedes Martinez, Chicago, IL *(Committee on Child Psychiatry)*
Michael Fuller McBride, Milwaukee, WI *(Committee on Public Education)*
Alan Newman, Little Rock, AR *(Committee on International Relations)*
Robert Rogan, Greenville, NC *(Committee on Occupational Psychiatry)*
Jennifer Felice Schreiber, New York, NY *(Committee on Medical Education)*
Roseanne State, Pacific Palisades, CA *(Committee on Therapy)*
Teresa M. Stathas, Columbia, SC *(Committee on Psychiatry and Religion)*
Lynelle Thomas, New Haven, CT *(Committee on Preventive Psychiatry)*
Anna Viltz, Houston, TX *(Committee on Human Sexuality)*
Kenneth William Wilson, New York, NY *(Committee on Mental Health Services)*
Larry Wissow, Baltimore, MD *(Committee on the Family)*

CONTRIBUTING MEMBERS

Gene Abroms, Ardmore, PA
Kenneth Z. Altshuler, Dallas, TX
Francis F. Barnes, Washington, DC
Spencer Bayles, Houston, TX
Elissa P. Benedek, Ann Arbor, MI
Renee L. Binder, San Francisco, CA
Mark Blotcky, Dallas, TX
H. Keith Brodie, Durham, NC
Charles M. Bryant, San Francisco, CA
Robert N. Butler, New York, NY
Eugene M. Caffey, Jr., Bowie, MD
Eric Caine, Rochester, NY
Robert J. Campbell, New York, NY
Sanford I. Cohen, Coral Gables, FL
Park Dietz, Newport Beach, CA
Robert E. Drake, Hanover, NH
James S. Eaton, Jr., Washington, DC
Lloyd C. Elam, Nashville, TN
Joseph T. English, New York, NY
Sherman C. Feinstein, Highland Park, IL
Paul Fink, Philadelphia, PA

Archie R. Foley, New York, NY
Henry J. Gault, Highland Park, IL
Richard K. Goodstein, Belle Mead, NJ
*Alexander Gralnick, Port Chester, NY
Joseph Green, Tucson, AZ
Milton Greenblatt, Sylmar, CA
Stanley I. Greenspan, Bethesda, MD
Jon E. Gudeman, Milwaukee, WI
William Hetznecker, Merion Station, PA
Johanna A. Hoffman, Scottsdale, AZ
Michael Kalogerakis, New York, NY
Edward J. Khantzian, Haverhill, MA
James A. Knight, New Orleans, LA
Othilda M. Krug, Cincinnati, OH
Judith Landau-Stanton, Rochester, NY
Alan I. Levenson, Tucson, AZ
Norman L. Loux, Sellersville, PA
Albert J. Lubin, Woodside, CA
John Mack, Chestnut Hill, MA
Alan A. McLean, Gig Harbor, WA
David Mendell, Houston, TX
Roy Menninger, Topeka, KS
Mary E. Mercer, Nyack, NY
Robert Michels, New York, NY
Sheldon Miller, Chicago, IL
Steven M. Mirin, Belmont, MA
Richard D. Morrill, Boston, MA
Joseph D. Noshpitz, Washington, DC
Mortimer Ostow, Bronx, NY
Bernard L. Pacella, New York, NY
Herbert Pardes, New York, NY
Norman L. Paul, Lexington, MA
Marvin E. Perkins, Salem, VA
George H. Pollock, Chicago, IL
Becky Potter, Tucson, AZ
Ann Price, Avon, CT
W. Donald Ross, Cincinnati, OH
Loren Roth, Pittsburgh, PA
Benson R. Snyder, Cambridge, MA

---

*Deceased.

David A. Soskis, Bala Cynwyd, PA
Jeffrey L. Speller, Cambridge, MA
Jeanne Spurlock, Washington, DC
Brandt F. Steele, Denver, CO
Terry Stein, East Lansing, MI
Alan A. Stone, Cambridge, MA
Perry C. Talkington, Dallas, TX
Bryce Templeton, Philadelphia, PA
Prescott W. Thompson, Portland, OR
John A. Turner, San Francisco, CA
Andrew S. Watson, Ann Arbor, MI
Paul Tyler Wilson, Bethesda, MD
Ann Marie Wolf-Schatz, Conshohocken, PA
Kent A. Zimmerman, Menlo Park, CA
Howard Zonana, New Haven, CT

LIFE MEMBERS

C. Knight Aldrich, Charlottesville, VA
Robert L. Arnstein, Hamden, CT
Walter E. Barton, Hartland, VT
Viola W. Bernard, New York, NY
Henry W. Brosin, Tucson, AZ
John Donnelly, Hartford, CT
Merrill T. Eaton, Omaha, NE
O. Spurgeon English, Narberth, PA
Stephen Fleck, New Haven, CT
Jerome Frank, Baltimore, MD
Robert S. Garber, Longboat Key, FL
Robert I. Gibson, Towson, MD
Margaret M. Lawrence, Pomona, NY
Jerry M. Lewis, Dallas, TX
Harold I. Lief, Philadelphia, PA
Earl Loomis, Augusta, GA
Judd Marmor, Los Angeles, CA
Herbert C. Modlin, Topeka, KS
John C. Nemiah, Hanover, NH
William C. Offenkrantz, Scottsdale, AZ
Perry Ottenberg, Philadelphia, PA
Mabel Ross, Sun City, AZ
Melvin Sabshin, Washington, DC

Julius Schreiber, Washington, DC
Robert E. Switzer, Dunn Loring, VA
Jack A. Wolford, Pittsburgh, PA
Henry H. Work, Bethesda, MD
Michael R. Zales, Tucson, AZ

BOARD OF DIRECTORS

Officers

President
Doyle I. Carson
777 Walter Reed #305
Garland, TX 75042

President-Elect
Malkah T. Notman
The Cambridge Hospital
54 Clark Road
Brookline, MA 02146

Secretary
Stephen C. Scheiber
ABPN
500 Lake Cook Road
Deerfield, IL 60015

Treasurer
Jack W. Bonner III
Behavioral Health Services
701 Grove Road
Greenville, SC 29605

Board Members
Gene Cohen
Leah Dickstein
Sally Severino
Joseph Westermeyer

Past Presidents

*William C. Menninger 1946–51
Jack R. Ewalt 1951–53
Walter E. Barton 1953–55
*Sol W. Ginsburg 1955–57
*Dana L.Farnsworth 1957–59
*Marion E. Kenworthy 1959–61
Henry W. Brosin 1961–63
*Leo H. Bartemeier 1963–65
Robert S. Garber 1965–67
Herbert C. Modlin 1967–69
John Donnelly 1969–71
GeorgeTarjan 1971–73
Judd Marmor 1973–75
John C. Nemiah 1975–77
Jack A. Wolford 1977–79
Robert W. Gibson 1979–81
*Jack Weinberg 1981–82
Henry H. Work 1982–85
Michael R. Zales 1985–87
Jerry M. Lewis 1987–89
Carolyn B. Robinowitz 1989–91
Allan Beigel 1991–93
John Schowalter 1993–95

PUBLICATIONS BOARD

Chairperson

Allan Beigel
P.O. Box 43460
Tucson, AZ 85733

David Adler
C. Knight Aldrich
Robert L. Arnstein
James Ellison
Ezra Griffith
Steve Katz
W. Walter Menninger

*Deceased.

Consultants

John C. Nemiah
Henry H. Work

Ex-Officio

Doyle Carson
John Schowalter

CONTRIBUTORS

Burroughs Wellcome Company
Glaxo Wellcome, Inc.
Edith F. Goldensohn
Jean Gumerson
Murel Foundation
Pharmacia/Upjohn Company
Phillips Foundation
Presbyterian Health Foundation
Wyeth-Ayerst Laboratories

GAP Publications

Alcoholism in the United States: Racial and Ethnic Considerations (GAP Report 141, 1996), Formulated by the Committee on Cultural Psychiatry

Adolescent Suicide (GAP Report 140, 1996), Formulated by the Committee on Adolescence

Mental Health in Remote Rural Developing Areas: Concepts and Cases (GAP Report 139, 1995), Formulated by the Committee on Therapeutic Care

Introduction to Occupational Psychiatry (GAP Report 138, 1994), Formulated by the Committee on Occupational Psychiatry

Forced Into Treatment: The Role of Coercion in Clinical Practice (GAP Report 137, 1994), Formulated by the Committee on Government Policy

Resident's Guide to Treatment of People With Chronic Mental Illness (GAP Report 136, 1993), Formulated by the Committee on Psychiatry and the Community

Caring for People With Physical Impairment: The Journey Back (GAP Report 135, 1992), Formulated by the Committee on Handicaps

Beyond Symptom Suppression: Improving Long-Term Outcomes of Schizophrenia (GAP Report 134, 1992), Formulated by the Committee on Psychopathology

---

*Title is out of print.

†Available from Books on Demand, University Microfilms International, 300 North Zeeb Road, Ann Arbor, MI 48106-1346 (800-521-0600, ext. 3492).

Psychotherapy in the Future (GAP Report 133, 1992), Formulated by the Committee on Therapy

Leaders and Followers: A Psychiatric Perspective on Religious Cults (GAP Report 132, 1992), Formulated by the Committee on Psychiatry and Religion

The Mental Health Professional and the Legal System (GAP Report 131, 1991), Formulated by the Committee on Psychiatry and the Law

***Psychotherapy With College Students** (GAP Report 130, 1990), Formulated by the Committee on the College Student

A Casebook in Psychiatric Ethics (GAP Report 129, 1990), Formulated by the Committee on Medical Education

***Suicide and Ethnicity in the United States** (GAP Report 128, 1989), Formulated by the Committee on Cultural Psychiatry

Psychiatric Prevention and the Family Life Cycle: Risk Reduction by Frontline Practitioners (GAP Report 127, 1989), Formulated by the Committee on Preventive Psychiatry

How Old Is Old Enough? The Ages of Rights and Responsibilities (GAP Report 126, 1989), Formulated by the Committee on Child Psychiatry

The Psychiatric Treatment of Alzheimer's Disease (GAP Report 125, 1988), Formulated by the Committee on Aging

Speaking Out for Psychiatry: A Handbook for Involvement With the Mass Media (GAP Report 124, 1987), Formulated by the Committee on Public Education

Us and Them: The Psychology of Ethnonationalism (GAP Report 123, 1987), Formulated by the Committee on International Relations

Psychiatry and Mental Health Professionals (GAP Report 122, 1987), Formulated by the Committee on Governmental Agencies

Interactive Fit: A Guide to Nonpsychotic Chronic Patients (GAP Report 121, 1987), Formulated by the Committee on Psychopathology

Teaching Psychotherapy in Contemporary Psychiatric Residency Training (GAP Report 120, 1986), Formulated by the Committee on Therapy

A Family Affair: Helping Families Cope With Mental Illness: A Guide for the Professions (GAP Report 119, 1986), Formulated by the Committee on Psychiatry and the Community

Crises of Adolescence—Teenage Pregnancy: Impact on Adolescent Development (GAP Report 118, 1986), Formulated by the Committee on Adolescence

The Family, the Patient, and the Psychiatric Hospital: Toward a New Model (GAP Report 117, 1985), Formulated by the Committee on Family

***Research and the Complex Causality of the Schizophrenias** (GAP Report 116, 1984), Formulated by the Committee on Research

***Friends and Lovers in the College Years** (GAP Report 115, 1983), Formulated by the Committee on the College Student

***Mental Health and Aging: Approaches to Curriculum Development** (GAP Report 114, 1983), Formulated by the Committee on Aging

Community Psychiatry: A Reappraisal (GAP Report 113, 1983), Formulated by the Committee on Psychiatry and the Community

The Child and Television Drama (GAP Report 112, 1982), Formulated by the Committee on Social Issues

***The Process of Child Therapy** (GAP Report 111, 1982), Formulated by the Committee on Child Psychiatry

The Positive Aspects of Long-Term Hospitalization in the Public Sector for Chronic Psychiatric Patients (GAP Report 110, 1982), Formulated by the Committee on Psychopathology

Job Loss—A Psychiatric Perspective (GAP Report 109, 1982), Formulated by the Committee on Psychiatry in Industry

A Survival Manual for Medical Students (GAP Report 108, 1982), Formulated by the Committee on Medical Education

INTERFACES: A Communication Casebook for Mental Health Decision Makers (GAP Report 107, 1981), Formulated by the Committee on Mental Health Services

***Divorce, Child Custody and the Family** (GAP Report 106, 1980), Formulated by the Committee on Family

***Mental Health and Primary Medical Care** (GAP Report 105, 1980), Formulated by the Committee on Preventive Psychiatry

Psychiatric Consultation in Mental Retardation (GAP Report 104, 1979), Formulated by the Committee on Mental Retardation

***Self-Involvement in the Middle East Conflict** (GAP Report 103, 1978), Formulated by the Committee on International Relations

The Chronic Mental Patient in the Community (GAP Report 102, 1978), Formulated by the Committee on Psychiatry and the Community

Power and Authority in Adolescence: The Origins and Resolutions of Intergenerational Conflict (GAP Report 101, 1978), Formulated by the Committee on Adolescence

***Psychotherapy and Its Financial Feasibility Within the National Health Care System** (GAP Report 100, 1978), Formulated by the Committee on Therapy

*†**What Price Compensation?** (GAP Report 99, 1977), Formulated by the Committee on Psychiatry in Industry

***Psychiatry and Sex Psychopath Legislation: The 30s to the 80s** (GAP Report 98, 1977), Formulated by the Committee on Psychiatry and Law

Mysticism: Spiritual Quest or Psychic Disorder? (GAP Report 97, 1976), Formulated by the Committee on Psychiatry and Religion

*†**Recertification: A Look at the Issues** (GAP Report 96, 1976), Formulated by the Ad hoc Committee on Recertification

*†**The Effect of the Method of Payment on Mental Health Care Practice** (GAP Report 95, 1975), Formulated by the Committee on Governmental Agencies

***The Psychiatrist and Public Welfare Agencies** (GAP Report 94, 1975), Formulated by the Committee on Psychiatry and the Community

***Pharmacotherapy and Psychotherapy: Paradoxes, Problems and Progress** (GAP Report 93, 1975), Formulated by the Committee on Research

***The Educated Woman: Prospects and Problems** (GAP Report 92, 1975), Formulated by the Committee on the College Student

*†**The Community Worker: A Response to Human Need** (GAP Report 91, 1974), Formulated by the Committee on Therapeutic Care

*†**Problems of Psychiatric Leadership** (GAP Report 90, 1974), Formulated by the Committee on Therapy

***Misuse of Psychiatry in the Criminal Courts: Competency to Stand Trial** (GAP Report 89, 1974), Formulated by the Committee on Psychiatry and Law

Assessment of Sexual Function: A Guide to Interviewing (GAP Report 88, 1973), Formulated by the Committee on Medical Education

From Diagnosis to Treatment: An Approach to Treatment Planning for the Emoti□onally Disturbed Child (GAP Report 87, 1973), Formulated by the Committee on Child Psychiatry

*†**Humane Reproduction** (GAP Report 86, 1973), Formulated by the Committee on Preventive Psychiatry

***The Welfare System and Mental Health** (GAP Report 85, 1973), Formulated by the Committee on Psychiatry and Social Work

*†**The Joys and Sorrows of Parenthood** (GAP Report 84, 1973), Formulated by the Committee on Public Education

***The VIP With Psychiatric Impairment** (GAP Report 83, 1973), Formulated by the Committee on Governmental Agencies

***Crisis in Child Mental Health: A Critical Assessment** (GAP Report 82, 1972), Formulated by the Ad hoc Committee

The Aged and Community Mental Health: A Guide to Program Development (GAP Report 81, 1971), Formulated by the Committee on Aging

***Drug Misuse: A Psychiatric View of a Modern Dilemma** (GAP Report 80, 1970), Formulated by the Committee on Mental Health Services

*†**Toward a Public Policy on Mental Health Care of the Elderly** (GAP Report 79, 1970), Formulated by the Committee on Aging

The Field of Family Therapy (GAP Report 78, 1970), Formulated by the Committee on Family

***Toward Therapeutic Care** (2nd Edition—No. 51 revised) (GAP Report 77, 1970), Formulated by the Committee on Therapeutic Care

***The Case History Method in the Study of Family Process** (GAP Report 76, 1970), Formulated by the Committee on Family

***The Right to Abortion: A Psychiatric View** (GAP Report 75, 1969), Formulated by the Committee on Psychiatry and Law

*†**The Psychiatrist and Public Issues** (GAP Report 74, 1969), Formulated by the Committee on International Relations

*†**Psychotherapy and the Dual Research Tradition** (GAP Report 73, 1969), Formulated by the Committee on Therapy

***Crisis in Psychiatric Hospitalization** (GAP Report 72, 1969), Formulated by the Committee on Therapeutic Care

***On Psychotherapy and Casework** (GAP Report 71, 1969), Formulated by the Committee on Psychiatry and Social Work

***The Nonpsychotic Alcoholic Patient and the Mental Hospital** (GAP Report 70, 1968), Formulated by the Committee on Mental Health Services

***The Dimensions of Community Psychiatry** (GAP Report 69, 1968), Formulated by the Committee on Preventive Psychiatry

***Normal Adolescence** (GAP Report 68, 1968), Formulated by the Committee on Adolescence

The Psychic Function of Religion in Mental Illness and Health (GAP Report 67, 1968), Formulated by the Committee on Psychiatry and Religion

***Mild Mental Retardation: A Growing Challenge to the Physician** (GAP Report 66, 1967), Formulated by the Committee on Mental Retardation

*†**The Recruitment and Training of the Research Psychiatrist** (GAP Report 65, 1967), Formulated by the Committee on Psychopathology

***Education for Community Psychiatry** (GAP Report 64, 1967), Formulated by the Committee on Medical Education

*†**Psychiatric Research and the Assessment of Change** (GAP Report 63, 1966), Formulated by the Committee on Research

*__Psychopathological Disorders in Childhood: Theoretical Considerations and a Proposed Classification__ (GAP Report 62, 1966), Formulated by the Committee on Child Psychiatry

*__Laws Governing Hospitalization of the Mentally Ill__ (GAP Report 61, 1966), Formulated by the Committee on Psychiatry and Law

*__Sex and the College Student__ (GAP Report 60, 1965), Formulated by the Committee on the College Student

*†__Psychiatry and the Aged: An Introductory Approach__ (GAP Report 59, 1965), Formulated by the Committee on Aging

*†__Medical Practice and Psychiatry: The Impact of Changing Demands__ (GAP Report 58, 1964), Formulated by the Committee on Public Education

Psychiatric Aspects of the Prevention of Nuclear War (GAP Report 57, 1964), Formulated by the Committee on Social Issues

*__Mental Retardation: A Family Crisis—The Therapeutic Role of the Physician__ (GAP Report 56, 1963), Formulated by the Committee on Mental Retardation

*__Public Relations: A Responsibility of the Mental Hospital Administrator__ (GAP Report 55, 1963), Formulated by the Committee on Hospitals

*__The Preclinical Teaching of Psychiatry__ (GAP Report 54, 1962), Formulated by the Committee on Medical Education

*__Psychiatrists as Teachers in Schools of Social Work__ (GAP Report 53, 1962), Formulated by the Committee on Psychiatry and Social Work

The College Experience: A Focus for Psychiatric Research (GAP Report 52, 1962), Formulated by the Committee on the College Student

*__Toward Therapeutic Care: A Guide for Those Who Work With the Mentally Ill__ (GAP Report 51, 1961), Formulated by the Committee on Therapeutic Care

*__Problems of Estimating Changes in Frequency of Mental Disorders__ (GAP Report 50, 1961), Formulated by the Committee on Preventive Psychiatry

*__Reports in Psychotherapy: Initial Interviews__ (GAP Report 49, 1961), Formulated by the Committee on Therapy

*__Psychiatry and Religion: Some Steps Toward Mutual Understanding and Usefulness__ (GAP Report 48, 1960), Formulated by the Committee on Psychiatry and Religion

*__Preventive Psychiatry in the Armed Forces: With Some Implications for Civilian Use__ (GAP Report 47, 1960), Formulated by the Committee on Governmental Agencies

*__Administration of the Public Psychiatric Hospital__ (GAP Report 46, 1960), Formulated by the Committee on Hospitals

*__Confidentiality and Privileged Communication in the Practice of Psychiatry__ (GAP Report 45, 1960), Formulated by the Committee on Psychiatry and Law

*__The Psychiatrist and His Roles in a Mental Health Association__ (GAP Report 44, 1960), Formulated by the Committee on Public Education

*__Basic Considerations in Mental Retardation: A Preliminary Report__ (GAP Report 43, 1959), Formulated by the Committee on Mental Retardation

*__Some Observations on Controls in Psychiatric Research__ (GAP Report 42, 1959), Formulated by the Committee on Research

*__Working Abroad: A Discussion of Psychological Attitudes and Adaptation in New Situations__ (GAP Report 41, 1958), Formulated by the Committee on International Relations

*__Small Group Teaching in Psychiatry for Medical Students__ (GAP Report 40, 1958), Formulated by the Committee on Medical Education

*__The Psychiatrist's Interest in Leisure-Time Activities__ (GAP Report 39, 1958), Formulated by the Committee on Public Education

The Diagnostic Process in Child Psychiatry (GAP Report 38, 1958), Formulated by the Committee on Child Psychiatry

*__Emotional Aspects of School Desegregation__ (an abbreviated and less technical version of Report No. 37) (GAP Report 37A, 1960), Formulated by the Committee on Social Issues

*__Psychiatric Aspects of School Desegregation__ (GAP Report 37, 1957), Formulated by the Committee on Social Issues

*__The Person With Epilepsy at Work__ (GAP Report 36, 1957), Formulated by the Committee on Psychiatry in Industry

*__The Psychiatrist in Mental Health Education: Suggestions on Collaboration With Teachers__ (GAP Report 35, 1956), Formulated by the Committee on Public Education

*__The Consultant Psychiatrist in a Family Service Agency__ (GAP Report 34, 1956), Formulated by the Committee on Psychiatry and Social Work

*__Therapeutic Use of the Self (A Concept for Teaching Patient Care)__ (GAP Report 33, 1955), Formulated by the Committee on Psychiatric Nursing

*__Considerations on Personality Development in College Students__ (GAP Report 32, 1955), Formulated by the Committee on the College Student

*__Trends and Issues in Psychiatric Residency Programs__ (GAP Report 31, 1955), Formulated by the Committee on Medical Education

*__Report on Homosexuality With Particular Emphasis on This Problem in Governmental Agencies__ (GAP Report 30, 1955), Formulated by the Committee on Governmental Agencies

*__The Psychiatrist in Mental Health Education__ (GAP Report 29, 1954), Formulated by the Committee on Public Education

*__The Use of Psychiatrists in Government in Relation to International Problems__ (GAP Report 28, 1954), Formulated by the Committee on International Relations

*__Integration and Conflict in Family Behavior__ (Reissued in 1968 as No. 27A) (GAP Report 27, 1954), Formulated by the Committee on Family

*__Criminal Responsibility and Psychiatric Expert Testimony__ (GAP Report 26, 1954), Formulated by the Committee on Psychiatry and Law

*__Collaborative Research in Psychopathology__ (GAP Report 25, 1954), Formulated by the Committee on Psychopathology

*__Control and Treatment of Tuberculosis in Mental Hospitals__ (GAP Report 24, 1954), Formulated by the Committee on Hospitals

*__Outline to Be Used as a Guide to the Evaluation of Treatment in a Public Psychiatric Hospital__ (GAP Report 23, 1953), Formulated by the Committee on Hospitals

*__The Psychiatric Nurse in the Mental Hospital__ (GAP Report 22, 1952), Formulated by the Committee on Psychiatric Nursing—Committee on Hospitals

*__The Contribution of Child Psychiatry to Pediatric Training and Practice__ (GAP Report 21, 1952), Formulated by the Committee on Child Psychiatry

*__The Application of Psychiatry to Industry__ (GAP Report 20, 1951), Formulated by the Committee on Psychiatry in Industry

*__Introduction to the Psychiatric Aspects of Civil Defense__ (GAP Report 19, 1951), Formulated by the Committee on Governmental Agencies

*__Promotion of Mental Health in the Primary and Secondary Schools: An Evaluation of Four Projects__ (GAP Report 18, 1951), Formulated by the Committee on Preventive Psychiatry

*__The Role of Psychiatrists in Colleges and Universities__ (GAP Report 17, 1951), Formulated by the Committee on Academic Education

*__Psychiatric Social Work in the Psychiatric Clinic__ (GAP Report 16, 1950), Formulated by the Committee on Psychiatry and Social Work

*__Revised Electro-Shock Therapy Report__ (GAP Report 15, 1950), Formulated by the Committee on Therapy

*__The Problem of the Aged Patient in the Public Psychiatric Hospital__ (GAP Report 14, 1950), Formulated by the Committee on Hospitals

*__The Social Responsibility of Psychiatry: A Statement of Orientation__ (GAP Report 13, 1950), Formulated by the Committee on Social Issues

*__Basic Concepts in Child Psychiatry__ (GAP Report 12, 1950), Formulated by the Committee on Child Psychiatry

*__The Position of Psychiatrists in the Field of International Relations__ (GAP Report 11, 1950), Formulated by the Committee on International Relations

*__Psychiatrically Deviated Sex Offenders__ (GAP Report 10, 1950), Formulated by the Committee on Forensic Psychiatry

*__The Relation of Clinical Psychology to Psychiatry__ (GAP Report 9, 1949), Formulated by the Committee on Clinical Psychology

*__An Outline for Evaluation of a Community Program in Mental Hygiene__ (GAP Report 8, 1949), Formulated by the Committee on Cooperation With Lay Groups

*__Statistics Pertinent to Psychiatry in the United States__ (GAP Report 7, 1949), Formulated by the Committee on Hospitals

*__Research on Prefrontal Lobotomy__ (GAP Report 6, 1948), Formulated by the Committee on Research

*__Public Psychiatric Hospitals__ (GAP Report 5, 1948), Formulated by the Committee on Hospitals

*__Commitment Procedures__ (GAP Report 4, 1948), Formulated by the Committee on Forensic Psychiatry

*__Report on Medical Education__ (GAP Report 3, 1948), Formulated by the Committee on Medical Education

*__The Psychiatric Social Worker in the Psychiatric Hospital__ (GAP Report 2, 1948), Formulated by the Committee on Psychiatric Social Work

*__Shock Therapy__ (GAP Report 1, 1947), Formulated by the Committee on Therapy

Index to GAP Publications #1–#80

Symposia Reports

The Right to Die: Decision and Decision Makers (S-12, 1973), Formulated by the Committee on Aging

*__Death and Dying: Attitudes of Patient and Doctor__ (S-11, 1965), Formulated by the Committee on Aging

*__Urban America and the Planning of Mental Health Services__ (S-10, 1964), Formulated by the Committee on Preventive Psychiatry

*__Pavlovian Conditioning and American Psychiatry__ (S-9, 1964), Formulated by the Committee on Research

*__Medical Uses of Hypnosis__ (S-8, 1962), Formulated by the Committee on Medical Education

*__Application of Psychiatric Insights to Cross-Cultural Communication__ (S-7, 1961), Formulated by the Committee on International Relations

*__The Psychological and Medical Aspects of the Use of Nuclear Energy__ (S-6, 1960), Formulated by the Committee on Social Issues

*__Some Considerations of Early Attempts in Cooperation Between Religion and Psychiatry__ (S-5, 1958), Formulated by the Committee on Psychiatry and Religion

*__Methods of Forceful Indoctrination: Observations and Interviews__ (S-4, 1957), Formulated by the Committee on Social Issues

*__Factors Used to Increase the Susceptibility of Individuals to Forceful Indoctrination: Observations and Experiment__ (S-3, 1956), Formulated by the Committee on Social Issues

*__Illustrative Strategies for Research in Psychopathology in Mental Health__ (S-2, 1956), Formulated by the Committee on Psychopathology

*__Considerations Regarding the Loyalty Oath as a Manifestation of Current Social Tension and Anxiety__ (S-1, 1954), Formulated by the Committee on Social Issues

Films

*__Discussion Guide to the Film__ (2, 1970)

*__A Nice Kid Like You__ (1, 1970)

Index

Page numbers printed in **boldface** *type refer to tables or figures.*

Index

Page numbers printed in **boldface** *type refer to tables or figures.*